ORTHOPAEDIC
PEARLS

ORTHOPAEDIC PEARLS

LEON S. BENSON, MD

Suburban Orthopaedic Associates, a division of
Illinois Bone & Joint Institute, Ltd.
Glenview, Illinois

Assistant Professor of Clinical Orthopaedic Surgery
Northwestern University Medical School
Chicago, Illinois

F. A. DAVIS COMPANY • Philadelphia

Printed in Canada

Last digit indicates print number: 10 9 8 7 6 5 4 3 2 1

Senior Medical Editor: Robert W. Reinhardt
Senior Developmental Editor: Bernice M. Wissler
Production Editor: Stephen D. Johnson
Cover Designer: Louis J. Forgione

As new scientific information becomes available through basic and clinical research, recommended treatments and drug therapies undergo changes. The author and publisher have done everything possible to make this book accurate, up to date, and in accord with accepted standards at the time of publication. The author, editors, and publisher are not responsible for errors or omissions or for consequences from application of the book, and make no warranty, expressed or implied, in regard to the contents of the book. Any practice described in this book should be applied by the reader in accordance with professional standards of care used in regard to the unique circumstances that may apply in each situation. The reader is advised always to check product information (package inserts) for changes and new information regarding dose and contraindications before administering any drug. Caution is especially urged when using new or infrequently ordered drugs.

Library of Congress Cataloging-in-Publication Data

Benson, Leon S., 1960–
    Orthopaedic pearls / Leon S. Benson.
        p.   cm.
    Includes bibliographical references and index.
    ISBN 0-8036-0185-9 (alk. paper)
    1. Orthopedics Handbooks, manuals, etc. I. Title.
    [DNLM: 1. Orthopedics Handbooks. 2. Orthopedic Equipment Handbooks. 3. Orthopedic Procedures Handbooks. WE 39 B474$_0$ 1999]
RD732.5.B46   1999
617.5--dc21
DNLM/DLC
for Library of Congress   99-14699
                                                                              CIP

To my wife, Karyn, and daughters Jessica and Rebecca, for allowing me to steal their time to work on this project;

To my brother Michael, for his incomparable leadership, intellect, and broad vision;

And to my parents, for teaching me the value of hard work (among everything else).

Preface

The main focus of this book is to serve as an aid to the "rookies"—medical students or brand-new residents who are just starting their orthopaedic housestaff experience. "How should I write post-op orders? What should I do when the floor nurse calls to report a patient with increasing pain? How should I handle the patient in the emergency room with a 'bimalleolar fracture'? How should I prepare for tomorrow's fracture conference? Is it my imagination, or does the OR scrub nurse hate me?"

These types of questions cannot be readily answered by standard textbooks and yet these are practical issues that the on-call houseofficer faces nightly. The novice orthopaedic staff person slowly accumulates a mammoth collection of multivolume fracture texts and surgical atlases in the call room; coat pockets are stuffed with fracture classifications and mnemonics scribbled on crumpled notecards, later to be lost in the laundry. Urgent runs are made upstairs to the call room between emergency room consults or operative cases in an attempt to "look up" the right answer. Unfortunately, the solution to the practical issue at hand for the on-call orthopaedic student or resident is never easy to locate in formal orthopaedic textbooks or research journals. Most of the hands-on information that the novice needs is traditionally taught informally, on a personal level, by a "big brother"–type mentor, either an empathetic attending or a more senior resident. *Orthopaedic Pearls* is a written diary of this kind of practical advice and allows the houseofficer to keep "big brother" in the oversized front coat pocket that is normally filled with useless penlights and plastic drug company goniometers.

Orthopaedic Pearls has been organized according to the different environments to which the student or resident will be exposed: the emergency room, the inpatient floor, the operating room, the office, and the conference room. The text can be read in a few hours and then kept handy for occasional reference as needed. It is *not* intended in any way to replace the formal study of comprehensive orthopaedic textbooks and journals. (An appropriate introductory reference list of such sources is given in Appendix F.) Orthopaedic science and clinical medicine comprise a constantly and rapidly expanding universe. There is no substitute for regular, intense study or the hard work that inherently characterizes good clinical care. And in addition to an organized reading curriculum, novices should read daily about the clinical situations they have personally encountered. Those particular cases will make text reading come alive and stick in their memory. By offering common sense and practical knowledge, this book may smooth over some of the bumps that occur in developing an orthopaedic compass.

Five people in particular deserve thanks for the preparation of this manuscript. Sandy Reinhardt, Bernice Wissler, Alison Kelley, and Samuel Rondinelli all have demonstrated superhuman patience with the vagaries of my writing schedule and have made significant editorial contributions that have greatly improved the finished product. Sherwood Benson, the "fourth musketeer," has been his usual invaluable self as an objective reviewer and source of inspiration for all difficult endeavors.

LEON S. BENSON, MD

Contents

1
PART

The Emergency Room

1
CHAPTER

General Principles

EMERGENCY ROOM CONDUCT

Because orthopaedic house staff spend a great deal of time in the emergency room (ER), it is important for them to develop a set of internalized responses that will help in successfully coping with this unique hospital environment. Although the ER often seems chaotic, it is the place where a great deal of orthopaedic learning and self-confidence will develop. Unfortunately, these "learning opportunities" occur at an unpredictable pace and often present themselves at the most inconvenient times. The frustration created by multiple phone calls, late-night consultations, and apparently disorganized patient presentations may challenge the temperament of even the most mature orthopaedic resident.

The following text presents some principles of ER conduct that I have found helpful. An extra amount of perspective and patience may be just what is needed to ensure that all parties, including the patient, the orthopaedic physician, and the ER staff, are happy with the orthopaedic consultation.

Your Behavior in the Emergency Room

In the ER, you are faced with a wide range of patients, from those who stubbed a toe to those whose leg was impaled by a telephone pole. There is something special about this environment that will add to your impatience, intolerance, frustration, fear, and exhaustion—setting you up to be less effective than you might otherwise be. These five *rules of conduct* will help you smoothly navigate your surroundings and provide patients with the best possible care.

1. **Stay calm at all times:** ER staff often sound or actually behave in an excited fashion. Either the injury they have just seen is dramatic, or the general busy atmosphere of the ER provides them with added stimulation. In any event, it will help your position to interact with everyone (whether patient, technician, attending physician, or nurse) in a calm, directed manner. Do not let the atmosphere cause you to unduly rush decision making, make unfounded assumptions, or bark orders or negative comments at anyone. A poised and organized demeanor quickly gains everyone's respect, and your job of treating the patient and functioning as a medical team member will be that much easier. Although these admonitions may appear obvious, the ER battlefield can launch even the most calm and organized person on the wrong course. Envision yourself as an ambassador from the "The United States of Orthopaedic Surgery," not as a disgruntled soldier forced to fight on foreign ground.

2. **Make no assumptions:** Do not assume that fractures, for example, are closed injuries until you examine the patient. When an ER intern has written in the chart, "neurovascular status within normal limits," this may mean very little. You need to examine and document the motor and sensory functions of every major peripheral nerve traveling through the injured zone and verify its status. I have never met an orthopaedic resident who was disappointed that the patient's injury was less complex than first described. However, the reverse scenario can be upsetting. Do not mistakenly *assume* that the radius fracture is a closed injury and that the median nerve is functioning just because someone from the ER phoned and said, "We have a Colles's fracture here for you." A better policy is to reserve judgment until *you* secure a thorough

history and physical exam *directly from the patient.* Use the help and input of those around you, but remember that you play a critical part in properly diagnosing the patient.

3. **Be independent:** Sometimes ER nurses are available to help you, and sometimes they are not. You will minimize time wasted and overall frustration if you work under the premise that you have to do everything yourself. Certainly, some tasks, such as putting on a long-leg cast, will be much easier if an assistant is there to help hold the leg. However, do not become one of those students or residents who must have everything "prepared" before seeing the patient. Learn the location of suture trays, tape, extra scissors, local anesthetic, syringes, bandages, and any other routine equipment. It may well be faster to grab this material yourself than to wait for someone else to get it for you. If your patient needs an intravenous (IV) line, do not hesitate to put in the line yourself if no one is present. You will save lots of time. If transporters are not available, wheel the patient to the radiology department for postcast films yourself. Fill out a pain medication prescription and discharge instructions while the patient is getting a postreduction x-ray. Everyone in the ER will be amazed not only at your speed in accomplishing care, but also at your initiative and good attitude. In doing all these tasks, you will probably get back to the call-room bed sooner. Furthermore, the more you try to do yourself, the more the nurses will be willing to offer you help spontaneously.

4. **Help others:** As you walk through the ER, you may be "curb sided." That is, someone will ask for you an unofficial opinion. Be friendly and generous with your time. Remember how much you appreciate it when someone gives you a little help. This also applies to the radiology technicians. They may be naturally apprehensive about getting a certain x-ray because it involves handling the broken bone and hurting the patient. Do not hesitate to run over to the radiology department and help the technician. The technician will be grateful, the patient will thank you, and you will get the exact radiographic view you want *the first time.*

5. **Keep a friendly exterior:** If you cannot smile, at least do not look foreboding and unapproachable. It may take considerable self-control, but not only will maintaining a pleasant exterior make you feel better, but everyone around you will be friendlier and more helpful. Sometimes you will be working under extreme strain and will depend on many others around you to be on your team. You will get into situations in which it seems as if the whole world is determined to irritate you. These irritations may come in the guise of a middle-of-the-night call to evaluate a "stubbed toe" or a long line of fractures waiting to be casted as soon as you get out of the operating room at 11 PM. Or, most certainly there will be the nurse who pokes her head into the trauma room while you are sewing up a hand laceration and announces, "Got another one for you," or "Hey doc, don't go anywhere." You know that the ER nurses and physicians have not injured these patients, nor have they solicited them to come to the hospital to disturb your 86 minutes of sleep. Stay focused on your No. 1 job, which is to care for patients in the best way possible. Furthermore, when you are about to explode at the ER intern who cannot describe an x-ray to your satisfaction, remember this: If everyone else knew how to read x-rays perfectly, how to put on casts, how to evaluate and manage extremity trauma, you would be out of a job. Take pride (silently) that you are an expert and that you can add the specialist's know-how in caring for these injuries. Every time you get that confused telephone description from a brand new ER intern, take a deep breath, smile, and say something like, "Thanks. I'll be right there."

THE ESSENTIAL ORTHOPAEDIC HISTORY AND PHYSICAL EXAM

Obtaining an accurate, complete history and physical exam (and documenting it concisely) is something you must be able to do effortlessly. The following guidelines show one way of documenting the necessary data. There are many other acceptable variations, and you will undoubtedly develop your own style and preferences.

History

1. **Name of patient, date, and time of encounter:** Do not skimp on carefully entering the date and time. Also write "Ortho History" at the top of the page. Many hospital medical record departments flag the chart for you to complete later if the information is not labeled as such.
2. **Chief complaint:** Examples include "wrist pain," "ankle pain," or "multiple trauma." The idea here is just to call attention to the main area of interest. Usually the patient's own words will suffice.
3. **History of present illness:** This is a two- to four-sentence summary of what is going on. Be brief. This is not like the history you used to write when you were a medical student on the internal medicine service. Be sure to include the following information:

   a. Patient's age, sex, and race
   b. Hand dominance
   c. Patient's occupation
   d. Date and possible time of injury
   e. Where injury occurred (sometimes crucial information in today's legal environment)
   f. For motor vehicle accidents, was patient:
      (1) Driver?
      (2) Restrained?
      (3) Thrown from a car?
      (4) In a high-energy or low-energy crash?
   g. For any trauma:
      (1) Did patient lose consciousness?
      (2) What preceded or precipitated trauma (i.e., did patient fall down, trip on a rug, have a stroke, or was he or she pushed down)?
      (3) Was it a high- or low-energy trauma (did patient fall downstairs versus being hit by a car)?
   h. What specific complaint does the patient volunteer?
      (1) Loss of soft-tissue integrity (i.e., bleeding)
      (2) Symptoms of neurovascular compromise

   Example: This patient is a 46-year-old, right-hand-dominant white female attorney who was struck by a car while she was crossing the street today at 10 AM. Patient did not lose consciousness and complains only of right-thigh pain and deformity. No numbness or tingling is present on that side; there is no neck or chest pain. Patient claimed that car was going approximately 25 mph.

4. **Medical history:** List items here such as hypertension, diabetes, sickle cell anemia, asthma, and so on. It can be helpful to ask, "When was the last time you were hospitalized?" Or, "Have you been in the hospital or ER anytime in the last 10 years?" This sometimes jogs the patient's memory, and some medical issues turn up. Also, some patients will deny any medical problems but then give you a long list of medications they are taking. Ask about the purpose of each medication; it is amazing what you will discover.
5. **Surgical history.**
6. **Orthopaedic history:** Ask particularly about previous implants and previous fractures (especially those relevant to current injury's location).
7. **Current medications.**
8. **Allergies.**
9. **Tobacco, alcohol, drug use.**
10. **Last meal:** What was consumed, how much, and exactly at what time?
11. **Last tetanus shot.**

Physical Exam

Focus your exam primarily on the extremities and spine, but also note the first five items that follow for the sake of completeness.

1. **General appearance:** Include relevant vital signs.
2. **Head and neck exam:** Note any obvious abnormalities, especially neck tenderness or abnormal curvature.
3. **Chest:** Assess for lung sounds and any abnormal spine curvature or tenderness.
4. **Heart:** Establish basic rhythm.
5. **Abdomen:** Auscultate for bowel sounds.
6. **Extremity exam:** Note the following items.

   a. Swelling
   b. Skeletal instability

   c. Location of tenderness
   d. Skin integrity: discoloration, wounds
   e. Motor function: test all peripheral nerves in region of injury and distal to it
   f. Sensibility: test all peripheral nerves in region of injury and distal to it
   g. Passive and active motion of joints proximal and distal to injury; also note if motion is painful.

7. **Spinal exam:**

   a. Swelling
   b. Location of tenderness
   c. Motor function and sensibility distal to level of interest
   d. Provocative tests: straight leg raise, etc.
   e. Reflexes

8. **Special issues for patients with multiple trauma:** Never assume that only one injury is present. For example, the same bone can be broken in two places several inches apart. The femur can be fractured in the midshaft, *and* the ipsilateral hip can be dislocated.

   a. Document motor and sensibility for *all* extremities
   b. Test range of motion and skeletal stability of all joints and bones in all extremities.
   c. Make sure the patient is fully undressed so that you do not miss anything (wounds, swelling, deformity, etc.). These patients are frequently unable to cooperate or communicate with you.

9. **Special issues for patients with spinal cord injury:**

   a. Treat these patients as you would patients with multiple trauma and spinal injury.
   b. Perform a rectal exam to determine injury level and prognosis. It is frequently overlooked or "deferred." Putting off this exam is completely unacceptable. You must document sphincter tone. Do this during your initial physical exam and get it over with.

MULTIPLE TRAUMA

Patients with multiple trauma require special attention because of the complexity associated with their care. As an orthopaedic resident, you will probably never function as the "team leader" in a multiple-trauma-care scenario, because this is traditionally performed by someone from general surgery (and usually the attending). However, there tend to be predictable pitfalls in managing patients with multiple trauma, and you can prevent these problems by understanding what issues often arise. Furthermore, occasionally a situation may arise in which you are the only one available to run a trauma resuscitation. In this case, knowing the protocol may save the patient's life.

Follow Protocol

Although each institution may have its own special style, the key issue is that *a plan must be followed*. Even though the general surgery service may be in charge, it is helpful for you to understand the overall sequence of events. Familiarize yourself with principles of fluid resuscitation and airway management. The protocol that I am familiar with is the Advanced Trauma Life Support program (Appendix A). Ideally, the orthopaedic resident will participate in the primary and secondary survey so that all of the patient's significant injuries (and consequently a care priority list) can be clarified. Certainly an open tibial fracture may not be more important than a ruptured spleen, but if all the injuries are noted before the patient goes to the operating room, total management is more efficient and organized. Many of the instances in which patients with multiple trauma "slip through the cracks" are related to a failure in following an organized care plan.

Examine the Patient Thoroughly

Patients with trauma should be disrobed so that injuries are not missed. A common mistake is not to examine the patient's back because he or she is lying on a backboard. Be sure to do the following in examining the patient:

1. Make sure that a rectal exam is performed; if the patient has a spinal cord injury or a significant pelvic fracture, you should do it.
2. Gently move all the extremity joints, from the shoulders to the fingertips, and from the hips to the toes.
3. Palpate every extremity long bone for crepitus, swelling, and instability.
4. Palpate and inspect the cervical spine and thoracolumbar spine. Even if the patient is unconscious or intubated, you will be able to identify most fractures or unstable joints.
5. Ensure that distal pulses are present and easily palpable.
6. Document the sensibility and motor status of all the major peripheral nerves.

The entire examination process usually takes only 2 minutes. Write down your findings immediately so that you do not forget and so that you will have an organized list of orthopaedic problems. Any area of abnormality on physical exam merits close attention; expand the detail of your physical exam and make sure that each injured region is appropriately x-rayed.

Obtain Appropriate X-rays

The basic series of films in any client with trauma includes chest x-ray, anteroposterior (AP) pelvis film, and a cervical (C) spine series (AP, lateral, and open-mouth views). The cervical films must clearly demonstrate C1 through T1 in two views. Make sure these films are obtained and scrutinized for any abnormality, because injuries to the neck, chest, or pelvis can easily result in the patient's death. The cervical spine almost always poses problems because the lower portion can be difficult to image. *Do not compromise.* If you cannot see the C7-T1 interval, pull down on the patient's arms to lower the shoulders while the film is repeated. If this does not work, get a "swimmer's view," in which one of the patient's arms is held forward flexed 180 degrees. If this does not work, consider alternative imaging such as tomograms or a computed tomography (CT) scan. No matter what you have to do, do not accept incomplete or poorly taken x-rays. Do not relinquish cervical spine immobilization until the necessary films are cleared as normal. If necessary, you may have to go with the patient to the radiology department to make sure the proper views are obtained (and obtained safely). It is faster to go help the radiology technician one time than it is to send the patient back to the radiology department three times until good films are obtained.

X-rays should be performed on any other part of the body that seems as if it might be injured. It is surprisingly easy to overlook significant fractures in patients with multiple trauma. Be sure to pursue a concentrated, thorough physical exam, and obtain films for any suspected swelling, instability, or tenderness. Do not be fooled by the presence of an IV line. These are frequently placed in extremities that have fractures or even directly over a broken bone.

The thoracolumbar spine and sacral spine are more difficult to examine than the extremities. I generally order an AP and lateral thoracolumbar spine series in almost every patient with multiple trauma.

One last word about x-rays. Double-check each x-ray to make sure that it is labeled correctly, not only with respect to the patient's name and date, but also as to which side (right or left) is represented on the film. Multiple-trauma scenarios tend to be chaotic and produce loads of paperwork and x-rays. Consider the following situation: A husband and wife are both injured in the same car crash, have similar injuries (bilateral tibia fractures), and only the last name is marked on the films. And by the way, all four sets of tibial films are marked "right." Whose tibia is whose? Which leg is which? You do not want to sort that out *after* you have arrived with one of the patients in the operating room.

Splint Extremity Fractures in the Emergency Room

Patients with trauma have a tendency to be whisked around the hospital, from the CT scan suite to the radiology department to the angiography lab and then to the operating room. You will probably have only one chance to efficiently place a splint on that fractured

General Principles   13

forearm, and that chance will be when you finish evaluating the patient in the ER. If no splint is placed then, more often than not, the patient is lifted by the fractured extremity when being transferred from one table to another. And you get to chase around the hospital, wasting time trying to find the patient so that you can place a splint (usually in an inconvenient or poorly controlled area, such as the radiology reception room). Some patients may even lie on an operating room table for hours with an unstable, unsplinted extremity. This predisposes them to potentially preventable conditions such as a neurapraxia, open fracture "in evolution," or a compartment syndrome. Do not let this be your patient.

Contact the Attending Surgeon Early

Patients with multiple trauma usually go to the operating room quickly, sometimes within 1 hour of their arrival. Assess the patient and the x-rays as soon as possible, and then call your attending surgeon. Some orthopaedic surgery attending physicians like to come to the hospital right away so that they can personally review the situation and plan the sequence of care or talk with the patient's family. Most attending physicians *do not* like to hear about the patient for the first time when the patient is actually on the operating room table undergoing a splenectomy.

ORTHOPAEDIC EMERGENCIES

Open Fractures

Open fractures require operative wound débridement within 6 hours or less from the time of injury. This is associated with significant reduction in infection rate and soft-tissue morbidity. In addition to the usual history, physical exam, and radiographic assessment, the following procedures will appropriately prepare your patient with open fracture for surgery:

1. Cover the wound with a sterile dressing. I prefer gauze soaked with Betadine.
2. Splint the extremity.

3. Make sure the patient is up to date on tetanus immunization or is given the appropriate tetanus prophylaxis in the ER. If this is not done in the ER, it has a tendency to be forgotten and never accomplished. The details of tetanus prophylaxis are discussed in Chapter 9.

4. Start antibiotic administration. Low-energy injuries merit a first-generation cephalosporin (cefazolin [Kefzol]). Patients with high-energy injuries should receive a cephalosporin and an aminoglycoside (Gentamicin). Severely contaminated wounds (farm injuries, wounds loaded with organic debris) should additionally be treated with penicillin.

5. Call your attending physician right away. It will be helpful to "grade" the fracture according to Gustilo and Anderson's system (Table 1–1).

6. Remember a key open-fracture principle: *It is probably more important to assess the degree of energy imparted to the limb rather than the exact size of the wound* in determining the character of an open injury. The energy transferred to the limb will characterize the injury's "personality" more accurately. The skin wound classification is simply a general guideline. Keep in mind, for example, that any fracture due to a high-velocity gunshot is classified as a grade III, even though the injury may have only a 1-cm entrance wound.

Cervical Spine Injuries

Treat patients with cervical spine injuries as if they were patients with multiple trauma. They usually are. Perform the full history, physical exam, and radiographic work-up. Do not forget a detailed neurologic exam and rectal exam. You must make sure that the cervical spine is fully immobilized throughout this process and remains so until definitive diagnosis is clear *and* treatment is rendered.

Changing Neurologic Examination

The issue here is to prevent the development of a permanent neurologic deficit. Loss of bowel or bladder control or rapid onset of any discrete motor or sensory

Table 1–1. GUSTILO-ANDERSON OPEN-FRACTURE CLASSIFICATION

Grade	Soft-Tissue Injury	Mechanism of Injury
I	Minimal, clean; wound ≤1 cm	Low energy
II	Moderate, some muscle damage, moderately contaminated; wound 2–10 cm	Moderate energy
III	High-energy or highly contaminated; wound >10 cm or open >8 h	High energy, e.g., high-velocity gunshot wounds, close-range shotgun wounds, barnyard injuries, segmental fractures
IIIA	Adequate soft-tissue coverage; complex reconstruction not usually required	
IIIB	Massive soft-tissue destruction and periosteal stripping; complex reconstruction required	
IIIC	Very severe loss of coverage associated with a repairable vascular injury	

loss should be a red flag. A few examples of non–trauma-related spinal cord compression include progressive infection (diskitis, osteomyelitis), encroachment by a tumor, or sudden disk herniation. These patients must be evaluated quickly, imaged appropriately (usually including emergency magnetic resonance imaging [MRI]) and then treated (emergency decompression, emergency radiation therapy, etc.).

Compartment Syndrome

Compartment syndrome occurs whenever the pressure within a closed anatomic compartment is high enough that microcirculation to tissue (especially muscle) in that compartment is compromised. After 4 to 6 hours, muscle starts to die and permanent loss ensues. The definitive treatment for compartment syndrome is to release the perimeter confining the space. The practical issue is making an early diagnosis and then reversing the process, either by loosening a tight cast, removing constricting bandages (or cast padding), or performing a fasciotomy. Following are examples of why intracompartmental pressures may rise to dangerous levels:

1. **Trauma:** Fracture hematoma is perhaps the No. 1 cause of compartment syndrome. Classic examples are tibial shaft or plateau fractures (leg compartment) and radial or ulnar shaft fractures (forearm compartment). Beware of any high-energy fracture types, such as segmental fractures. Compartment syndrome can occur just about anywhere, including the thigh, the hand, and the foot.
2. **Infection:** Accumulation of pus will drive intra-compartmental pressures up.
3. **Burns:** Tremendous associated soft-tissue edema will produce high compartmental pressures. Circumferential eschars can also act to constrict the extremity and worsen distal swelling.
4. **Limb compression:** Believe it or not, continued compression of a limb, such as sleeping on it for 8 hours, can reduce local blood flow to levels that will not support the metabolic demands of muscle and nerve tissue. Most people shift around when they sleep and no problems occur. However, intoxicated or drugged individuals may be motionless for up to 12 hours and then present with a swollen, tense, and tender extremity. Consider compartment syndrome. Beware of the patient who is still intoxicated or uncooperative; you may not have the benefit of tenderness in helping with the diagnosis.

The clinical findings in compartment syndrome include:

- Pain at rest
- Paresthesias
- Soft-tissue tenseness

• Pain with passive motion of joints distal to the compartment

Pain out of proportion to the patient's situation is an ominous sign. Traditional texts refer to the "five Ps" of diagnosis: *p*ain, *p*allor, *p*aralysis, *p*aresthesias, and *p*ulselessness. Paralysis can be a late finding, however, and pulselessness is very unreliable. Distal pulses are usually intact because, although capillary-level circulation will be compromised, rarely is enough pressure present to initially stop blood flow in the major peripheral vessels. Pain is the earliest and most reliable indicator. Particularly note if the pain is very severe, does not respond well to immobilization or pain medication, and tends to progressively worsen (described as a "crescendo" pattern).

The definitive method of diagnosing compartment syndrome is by measuring compartment pressures. This is detailed in Appendix B. A good rule to follow is *any time you even think a compartment syndrome may be present, measure pressures.* Compartment pressure greater than 40 mm Hg (or within 30 mm of the diastolic blood pressure) should prompt intervention. If measured pressures are not high enough to justify fasciotomy, make sure nothing is constricting the extremity and follow the patient closely. I recommend personally reexamining the patient every hour until you are certain that no progression is occurring.

It can be difficult to distinguish compartment syndrome from fracture pain, ischemia, or nerve injury. *Fracture pain* can be severe but is usually well controlled or at least improved with immobilization. Elevate the limb so that the injured area is even with the heart. (A lower level will increase venous pooling; if the limb is higher it may decrease arterial inflow.) Proper elevation sometimes requires three or four pillows under the leg to prop it up level with the reclining patient's chest. Loosen tight casts by either splitting or bivalving them with a cast saw. Better to lose the fracture reduction than to compromise limb circulation. Sometimes you may even have to tear the cast padding open to relieve pressure caused by fracture swelling. Cast padding can become remarkably tight; after you split the cast, you can then use your fingers to tear a longitudinal defect in the padding. Any fracture pain that does not respond promptly to immobilization, elevation, cast splitting, and modest oral pain medication should be investigated aggressively to rule out an incipient compartment syndrome.

With *ischemic pain,* the area distal to the blockage is not usually tense. Palpation of a compartment syndrome region typically demonstrates dramatic soft-tissue tension that is exquisitely tender to slight compression.

With *nerve injury,* paralysis and paresthesia are present, but these injuries are not usually characterized by pain or soft-tissue tension.

Joint Dislocation

Any traumatically dislocated joint should be reduced as soon as possible. Prolonged dislocation (even more than 30 minutes) will stretch the skin and surrounding soft-tissue envelope, increasing the likelihood of skin breakdown and neurovascular compromise. Furthermore, some dislocations may actually compromise the viability of the bone dislocated (the femoral head in a hip dislocation). Some practical points follow:

1. **Always check postreduction films** and make sure that you have orthogonal views (perpendicular to each other, such as an AP and lateral). It is easy to be fooled by a single AP view of the hip. For example, a posterior hip dislocation may look perfectly reduced on an AP film, but the lateral film will show what is happening. Never assume that you have reduced the joint until you can prove it with films.
2. **If you cannot easily reduce a joint, get help:** Do not flail away 10 times trying to yank the bone back into place. You will exhaust yourself, inflict great pain on the patient, and possibly injure the bone and soft tissues. Help may take the form of another person to stabilize the patient, or even better, a little bit of IV sedation. Study the films and think about how the bone came out of place; this will help you logically devise your reduction maneuver. You will be called to the ER to reduce a shoulder that the ER staff could not. Even if the ER physicians are bigger or stronger than you, do not worry. Joint reduction

tends to be a *finesse* maneuver, not one of great strength. Be attentive to the "preconditions" for joint reduction and you will succeed with surprising ease. Carefully sedate the patient, calmly plan the best reduction maneuver, secure the patient's body with an assistant, and eliminate any observers.

3. **Prosthetic dislocations are a special case:** A common situation is the dislocated total hip arthroplasty. You may choose to attempt reduction first, although some hip surgeons prefer to be notified right away because they have their own protocol for managing these patients. In some cases, closed reduction is not possible owing to loosening and shifting of the acetabular component, or dissociation of a polyethylene liner from the cup. Study the films carefully before you attempt reduction. In cases of component loosening, reduction may require operative intervention and even revision arthroplasty.

Septic Flexor Tenosynovitis

Infection in the hand flexor tendon space can be catastrophic. The sublimus and profundus flexor tendons fit together precisely and glide through the digital pulley system with very little clearance. Infection in this zone will quickly produce scarring and adhesions that can permanently compromise tendon function. Infection will also start to liquefy the tendon itself, producing irreparable damage. The standard treatment for a septic flexor tenosynovitis is immediate operative irrigation and drainage (in addition to antibiotics). Septic flexor tenosynovitis is reviewed in more detail in Chapter 9.

Gas Gangrene

Gas gangrene is one of several histotoxic infections that can quickly kill a patient. Other potentially life-threatening, fast-acting infectious processes are anaerobic cellulitis, streptococcal myonecrosis, and toxic shock syndrome. Please refer to Chapter 9 for discussion of these dangerous infections.

CASTS AND SPLINTS

The application of casts and splints will consume a large part of the orthopaedic resident's time in the ER. Unfortunately, cast application is a "hands-on" skill, and there is no substitute for experience. The more casts you apply, the better you will get. Do not be discouraged by the peculiar appearance of your first 25 casts (or by how long it takes you to apply them). Practice reliably yields better-fitting casts and faster application. Clarification of the following issues will help you master good casting skills.

Cast or Splint?

The decision to cast or to splint depends on the type of fracture, its location, patient issues, and personal preference. For example, I prefer to place freshly reduced distal radial fractures in a cast and then split the cast to allow for swelling. Some surgeons may prefer the "Charnley splint," which is an anterior and posterior plaster splint. These splints probably accomplish the same goal as casting, although it is my opinion that a cast more reliably holds the fracture reduction. However, because casts are rigid, circumferential bandages, be careful to split them with a cast saw so that acute swelling can be accommodated. If severe swelling is predictable, a splint for the immediate postinjury period is probably safer. The following are special considerations regarding casting or splinting:

- In *children with a torus-type fracture of the distal radius,* a splint would be adequate immobilization, except that most children will destroy or remove a splint within 24 hours. A cast is better here.
- A *reduced elbow dislocation* is better treated with a long-arm posterior mold than a cast. The mold better accommodates swelling. Furthermore, motion of the elbow typically commences within 1 or 2 weeks, so why place a long-arm cast, which will have to removed within several days?
- Many *hand fractures* are better immobilized by taking strips of plaster and constructing a custom-formed splint one piece at a time. Attempting to

apply a cast around the digital web spaces can be very difficult. As you gain experience, you learn how to juggle these factors and the choice of device will become second nature and subject to your preferences.

Plaster or Fiberglass?

Plaster is better for holding reduction of a fresh fracture. It can be molded more intricately and can be made to fit literally like a glove. It is messier, however, and generally takes longer to dry (sometimes up to 24 hours to really harden).

Fiberglass is more wear resistant and stronger than plaster (fiberglass will not crack). It is also about one-third lighter than plaster. I think of fiberglass more as a "protective" cast material that must weather many weeks of wear, whereas plaster is better to hold a broken bone in position for the first few weeks of healing.

You can mix materials to get the best out of each. Sometimes an initial layer of plaster can be used to mold to the extremity, and then an outer coat of fiberglass is applied to add strength. I often will change distal radial fractures from plaster to fiberglass at about 3 weeks.

Types of Plaster

Once you gain some experience in applying casts, you will want to use the fastest-setting plaster available. Using warm water will speed the setup time of either plaster or fiberglass. Just be sure *not* to use hot water, or you can easily burn the patient's skin. Room temperature water is about right—certainly no warmer.

Chaston (Melville, New York) and Johnson & Johnson both manufacture a popular brand of plaster. Chaston supplies Gypsona II, which is creamy and easy to mold. It can be quite weak, however, unless you apply lots of it. Specialist, Johnson & Johnson's plaster bandage, is more like wet cardboard when you first apply it. This is because most of the good plaster content is in the center of the roll. Be sure to use the whole roll and then rub the plaster vigorously. It blends quite nicely. Johnson & Johnson's plaster is extremely strong.

For forearm casts, I prefer to use a roll or two of Gypsona II and then apply an outer coat of Johnson & Johnson's to add strength and durability.

Rolling Plaster and Fiberglass

Narrower rolls are easier to use when turning corners, so 2- and 3-inch widths are good for the hand and wrist. Wider rolls save time in application and are commonly used proximal to the wrist and foot. When rolling cast material (or padding), overlap each revolution by about 50 percent. When applying a long-arm or long-leg cast, it is sometimes easier to apply the distal half first, let it partially harden so that the fracture is held, and then secondarily apply the upper portion of the cast. Make sure that you "bond" the two halves together well by running some cast rolls the entire length of the extremity; otherwise, the cast tends to crack and break at the junction site between the two halves. Also, be sure that you have adequate padding at the halfway point; it is easy to mistakenly "underpad" this area. If this occurs, it can be hard to add padding here once the distal half of the cast dries.

Long-leg Casts

Tremendous strength can be gained by incorporating an "anterior bar." This is especially useful for long-leg casts in large patients. Take five thicknesses of 5- by 30-inch plaster splints, bunch them together longitudinally, and apply them as an anterior 3-inch-wide bar down the length of the cast, centered about the patella. Then roll a last layer of plaster, incorporate this bar and finish off the cast. The anterior bar makes cracking the cast at the knee virtually impossible once it dries.

When the Cast Starts to Dry

You have several "golden" minutes to mold and shape its contour as the cast begins to dry. This period is often heralded by the cast developing a dull, pasty look to its exterior. Rubbing the cast vigorously tends to blend all of the individual cast-tape revolutions together and yield a stronger, more coherent final product. It will also look better. Be careful not to press too hard with your fingertips to avoid producing any pressure points in the cast. Areas that warrant particular attention include bony prominences such as the heel.

When molding plaster, it is safer to use the flat of your hand to prevent any sharp indentations in the cast. An apparently harmless indentation caused by pressure from your single fingertip can produce a prominence inside the cast and actually generate skin breakdown and a large, infected ulceration. Be particularly careful with patients who have delicate skin, such as elderly people or those on chronic steroid medication.

Padding

How much cast padding to use really depends on where the cast is being applied and for what reason. Padding should be "beefed up" around bony prominences (e.g., olecranon, malleoli) and near a fracture site (anticipate swelling). However, too much padding makes the cast fit poorly. Usually two layers is enough for most of the cast, adding more in special areas. As you roll padding (or plaster), generally overlap each revolution by about 50 percent. Remember that "Webril" is a cottony padding that is appropriate for plaster, whereas fiberglass casts require special synthetic cast padding designed specifically for fiberglass.

Stockinet

Stockinet is a sock-type liner that adds to the cast's appearance because you can turn it over and tuck in the edges of the cast. Some surgeons prefer to use full-length stockinet (rather than just at the proximal and distal ends of the cast) because they believe it is less likely to wrinkle or shift. If you use full-length stockinet, cut a slot in areas that cross flexion creases so that no bunching occurs. Also, be careful not to stretch the material while applying (this produces a stockinet abrasion, obvious when the cast comes off).

Cast Saw

Cast saws have a vibrating blade. Total excursion on the blade is only about 3 mm, even though it looks and sounds as though it is a circular saw. Theoretically, the limited travel on the saw-blade teeth will not effectively cut any material that stretches, so it cuts nicely through plaster but not cast padding or skin. Explaining this to patients (especially children) and warning them about the noise will greatly reduce their anxiety. Do not demonstrate the safety of the saw by touching the running blade on your palm. If pressed with any pressure at all, you will cut yourself and bleed in front of the patient. The saw is actually quite safe, but it is easy to cut skin by dragging the blade.

Splitting Technique

Proper sawing technique involves pressing the saw into the cast until it pops through and then removing it and making another contiguous cut about 2 inches away. Cutting a cast is more like making 15 contiguous line segments in the cast, all connected. Dragging the saw through the cast will reliably cut or abrade skin. Extreme care should be used when cutting a cast off of a baby or an older person because their skin is so fragile.

Holding the cast saw securely is the key point in using the saw safely and efficiently. Use your dominant hand to grip the neck of the saw and place the thumb of that hand onto the cast surface. Pressure from your thumb now controls the depth of each cut. You can also additionally use your nondominant hand to bridge the distance between the saw and the cast to add additional control. As you feel the blade penetrate the inner side of the cast material, back out immediately.

As the cast saw blade cuts, it heats up. This is especially true when cutting through fiberglass. Pause for a few seconds between each saw application to let the blade cool down. When a patient jumps while a cast is being cut, it is usually because heat has conducted though the padding and the patient feels a sharp jolt of pain. Although the patient will think his skin has been nicked, actually the problem usually is an overheated saw blade getting near the skin surface.

For any cast applied within 5 days of an injury, it is prudent to split the cast with a cast saw before the patient leaves the ER. This allows the cast to open slightly and accommodate swelling. It often saves a midnight phone call or return trip to the ER.

Most casts can be split by cutting a longitudinal slot in whatever surface is conveniently exposed (dorsal in the upper extremity, anterior in the lower extremity). The cut should run the entire length of the cast. Furthermore, simply cutting once with the cast saw is not adequate. It is better to make two parallel longitudinal cuts 5 mm apart and then remove this 5-mm strip of material. Next, use a cast spreader to "crack" open the cast a tiny bit. This will not compromise fracture reduction and tends to stretch the padding a little bit so the cast can indeed expand if swelling occurs.

Also, note that it is much more difficult to properly split a cast if it is still very wet. Get postreduction films on your patient, write up their ER sheet, fill out a pain medication prescription, finish a discharge form, review the films with them, discuss follow-up and care instructions, and *then* split the cast. By then, even plaster will be dry enough to allow proper splitting.

Bivalving

Bivalving a cast involves making two longitudinal cuts with a saw, each 180 degrees apart. This creates two equal parts of the cast and relieves even more pressure than making a single cut. Bivalving, however, compromises the cast's structural integrity more than splitting. Some surgeons prefer to bivalve a cast and then loosely wrap an elastic bandage or tape around it to help hold it together in its widened state.

Inserting a Window

Windowing a cast involves cutting out a rectangular portion, usually to allow inspection of a wound or surgical incision. When a cast is applied over a wound, many surgeons will mark the cast directly over the wound so that it is easy to place a cast window later. The key point with creating windows is to replace the window segment carefully after the wound has been examined and the dressing changed. Failing to replace a cast segment will allow swelling to occur through the cast defect, producing window edema. Once this edema starts, it is often impossible to remedy without replacing the entire cast. So if you window a cast, do not throw out that "little piece" you excise with the cast saw. Inspect the wound and then replace the window segment carefully by taping it back in place securely.

Prepping the Skin

When severe injuries are going to be immobilized by a cast or splint (even temporarily), the underlying skin should first be prepped with an antiseptic, such as Betadine. Especially if skin blistering is likely, it is prudent to prep the skin so that if a blister breaks inside the cast, bacterial contamination of the blister is reduced.

Patient Instructions

Provide the patient with guidelines or instructions for home cast care, as follows:

1. Inform the patient that if there are any problems with the cast (e.g., too tight, too loose, severe pain, swelling, tingling, burning, numbness, coldness), they must return to the ER or call their doctor immediately.
2. Proper elevation of the extremity may provide better pain relief than narcotic pain medication (and with less side effects).
3. All casts must be kept dry. Although fiberglass cast tape is waterproof, the underlying padding is not and will soak up water like a sponge, forcing a cast change. Although some newer cast padding is available that is waterproof, I use it only rarely. It is difficult to apply and does not fit very well. Furthermore, I believe it tends to encourage the wrong behavior for patients with fractures. Showering can be accomplished by wrapping a towel around the proximal end of the cast and then covering the extremity with a plastic bag secured with a large rubber band.
4. Patients should be instructed not to scratch under

a cast (with a pen, for example) because it is easy to cut or abrade the skin, and ulcerations or infection can ensue. I tell patients who worry about itching to scratch the opposite extremity in the same place on which they feel the casted side itch. I do not know if it really works, but many patients have told me it makes them forget about the itch. The best way to prevent itching is not to stretch stockinette (if it is used) and to clean and dry the skin before the cast is applied.

THE PEDIATRIC PATIENT

Managing pediatric patients in the ER sometimes requires a slightly different approach than you use with adult patients. Most junior orthopaedic residents dread dealing with pediatric patients. Typically, they feel this way for two reasons: (1) administering an anesthetic to the fracture site (or to the whole patient) may be more complicated, and (2) extraneous observers (concerned parents) ask questions, scrutinize every move, and require lengthy explanations during the treatment process. Fortunately, these issues can be easily dealt with as long as you are prepared.

Basic anesthetic techniques for children can be similar to those for adults. For example, many fractures will do well with a simple hematoma block. The problem occurs when having to inject a child for anything, whether it be a hematoma block or simply placing an IV line. Once children start to cry, they generally cry vigorously and continuously as long as you are present. They know that you represent "treatment," and treatment may mean more needles and pain. The crying will serve to unnerve and distract you, and in most cases, it stimulates a more protective, doubtful attitude from the parents. Note the following simple suggestions.

When First Called

Try to have the ER staff prepare the pediatric patient for you before you arrive. Find out what type of fracture is present, and decide right then if you want an IV line, or intramuscular administration of sedation, or both. If you do, ask if the ER staff can place the line and/or sedate the child. Although you should be willing to do these things yourself in the name of being independent, most ER nurses will be happy to accomplish these tasks before you arrive. The great benefit is that you personally have been separated from details that most children dislike. Your slate, so to speak, is still clean. In the eyes of both parents and child, you have so far done nothing painful or unpleasant. Furthermore, a little bit of sedation will go a long way to relax the patient, and when you first introduce yourself, no one will be hysterical.

Explanation to Parents

Clearly explain to the parents what type of injury is present and what you need to do right now. Keep this discussion reasonably brief and convey confidence. Reviewing the x-rays before you go into the room is helpful. If fracture manipulation is required, you may next ask the parents to retreat to the waiting room until you are finished. Children exhibit more distress if their parents are present. If the parents refuse to leave, do not make this a big issue. If additional family members are present, however, insist that they leave. I try to allow only one parent in the room for any ER procedure; more than that creates unacceptable distraction for both patient and physician. Make sure the family retreats away from the treatment room. Standing outside the door is worse than being in the room. Direct them to the waiting room or the hospital cafeteria.

Manipulating the Fracture

When it comes time to manipulate the fracture or do anything painful, be reasonably honest with the child if you are asked, "Will it hurt?" However, minimize the time between announcing a fracture manipulation and actually performing one. Children will start to cry the minute you tell them that something painful might be happening soon. Do not then delay 15 minutes. Tell them you need to move the bone back in position, and then do it within 30 seconds. Everyone will be happier.

Child Abuse Injuries

Child abuse is faced by physicians far more than is commonly thought and occurs with similar frequency throughout a wide spectrum of socioeconomic backgrounds. Beyond the moral imperatives of reporting abuse, the orthopaedic surgeon has a legal obligation to report suspected child abuse. As a resident, notify your attending physician immediately if you are suspicious. It is also prudent to discreetly discuss details of the history and physical findings with the ER attending. Usually, the ER attending physician, the orthopaedic attending physician, or attending pediatrician (or some combination thereof) will make the decision to contact the appropriate authorities. A victim of suspected child abuse should be admitted to the hospital, both for the child's own protection as well as to pursue appropriate medical work-up (e.g., skeletal survey, bone scan) and treatment (e.g., for burns, fractures).

The following list highlights issues that may suggest incidents of child abuse.

- A history of injury that does not correlate with the physical findings
- Different injury histories from different family members
- Multiple injuries, especially when they seem to be in different stages of healing
- Skin wounds or burns
- Fractures of the ribs, long bones, or skull when other suspicious signs are present
- Spiral or oblique long-bone fractures in the lower extremities of children who are not yet ambulatory; remember that 50 percent of long-bone fractures in children younger than 1 year and 80 percent in infants younger than 6 months are associated with child abuse
- Posterior rib fractures
- Metaphyseal corner fractures in the lower-extremity long bones of children who are not yet ambulatory

PAPERWORK IN THE
EMERGENCY ROOM

Carefully document everything that you do. This is not only a legal issue, but also a matter of safety and quality of care.

Admission

If a patient is being admitted, write out a history and physical findings that have all the necessary information. However, if you send someone home from the ER, be sure to write a small note that summarizes what care has been administered. I prefer to draw a 4-inch-wide box on the ER record and write "Ortho" at the top. If the history has already been documented by the ER staff on that page, you can write, "History: as above." Then within the box document the pertinent physical findings, especially noting skin integrity, neurovascular status, and any deformity. Summarize the radiographic findings, and then note what you did to the patient. "1 percent Xylocaine (without epinephrine) hematoma block administered sterilely to fracture site; closed reduction performed and long-arm cast applied. Postreduction films obtained." Also document that you split the cast and explained follow-up and care instructions to the patient. Write as clearly as you can so that someone else reviewing the record 2 months later could make sense of your note.

Discharge Instruction Sheet

Fill out a discharge instruction sheet, and even better, go over it with the patient and family and have him or her sign it. This will endear you to the ER nurses, because you have saved them the trouble of "signing out" the patient. Patients also are favorably impressed if you take a little extra time to address their questions personally. Do not, however, send the patient home at this point. Just tell the nurse that the patient is ready to leave and that the discharge form is signed. The nurse will still want to talk to the patient and make sure that everything is in order. On the discharge instruction sheet, indicate a phone number that the patient should call to make a follow-up appointment and also who to call if an emergency arises. Characterize for the patient what constitutes an emergency. Indicate that severe pain or swelling, numbness, tingling, and discoloration are issues that should be evaluated immediately by a physician. It is also helpful to write some extra tips, like "Keep wrist elevated" and "Keep cast dry."

Pain Medication Prescription

The prescription for pain medication is the last bit of usual paperwork. Never walk around with signed, completed prescriptions that require only a patient's name. These will not save you any significant time and only get you into serious trouble because they are invariably misplaced or stolen.

The type of pain medication you will prescribe depends on the type of injury and your personal preference. I generally stick with one or two medications to keep my life simple. Hydrocodone (Vicodin) is a good choice for many fractures, as is acetaminophen (Tylenol No. 3 [with codeine]). I try to stay away from more powerful narcotics, such as oxycodone (Percocet), because I do not believe that most outpatients need this amount of narcotic (and it can be very addictive). For a typical fracture (distal radius), I will usually write for about 30 pain pills so that the patient will have enough for the first 4 or 5 days. I also prefer to indicate "No refills" because if the patient needs more pain medication, I like to know about it. All of the medication you prescribe will produce side effects eventually, and it is probably better to use a small amount of narcotic combined with physical measures, such as ice and elevation. Elevating the extremity may do more to reduce pain and swelling than any amount of medication.

TELEPHONING THE ORTHOPAEDIC ATTENDING PHYSICIAN

Proper telephone manner might seem to be a trivial point, but many attending physicians will unavoidably judge orthopaedic residents and students by their telephone savvy. The fundamental rule is "be organized." Just before you start dialing, grab the patient's chart, place it in front of you, and briefly review it. It is embarrassing when you cannot quickly recite the patient's name, age, or injured side when asked on the phone. Even though you may have just spent 10 minutes talking to the patient, you will be surprised how hard it is to remember their name or age. Having the chart available will also allow you to look up anything else you might be asked, like lab results, the patient's address, or insurance carrier.

When you first start talking to the attending physician, identify yourself as one of the orthopaedic residents, especially if you are calling in the middle of the night. Many people are not completely alert when they first awake. Then, in just a few sentences, explain the situation. Include the patient's age, occupation, mechanism of injury, date and approximate time of injury, pertinent physical findings, and radiographic findings. I prefer to announce in the first few words the actual injury. Then review the situation details. Nothing can be more frustrating than hearing a long, mostly irrelevant description of some incident, with the actual injury being withheld as though it is the big surprise in a suspense movie. Certainly, in cases where the attending physician has to come to the hospital immediately (open fracture, etc.), indicate this clearly at the beginning of your phone call. To illustrate these points, two scenarios are noted below. The orthopaedic resident is calling his attending about an elderly man with a hip fracture. It is 2 AM.

Scenario A

Attending: Hello?
Resident: Hey, how are ya! It's me.
A: Hello? Who is this?
R: It's one of the boys. How's it going?
A: Who is this?
R: It's Bob in ER. Got one for you.
A: What's going on?
R: Got a nice guy here who fell. You should see his films!
A: What's wrong with him?

R: His name is John. Used to own a record store. Anyway, I had to really sedate him.
A: What's wrong with him?
R: Probably has a hip fracture. Don't have all the films yet. No—wait a minute. Here they are. Yup, it's the hip all right.
A: What kind of fracture?
R: Pretty bad. We'll have to get more films to tell for sure . . .

This type of phone call can go on for another 5 minutes before the attending physician has a clear picture of the situation. The resident may certainly be enthusiastic and intelligent, but he has not conveyed these qualities over the telephone.

Scenario B

Attending: Hello?
Resident: Hi, Dr. Jones. It's Bob Smith, the orthopaedic resident. I'm in Community Hospital's ER.
A: What's up?
R: I have an elderly gentleman here with a closed, left, two-part intertrochanteric hip fracture. The patient's name is John Doe, and he is an 82-year-old retired businessman who slipped on a rug at home 2 hours ago, falling onto his side. He has no other relevant medical problems and is an independent ambulator who lives alone.
A: Sounds like he needs to be admitted and prepared for surgery. Any other injuries?
R: No other injuries. We've got all his labs already. I put a call in to his medical attending who's going to see him in the morning. I added the patient to the OR schedule for tomorrow afternoon.
A: Hey thanks, Bob. See you in the morning.

Scenario B illustrates a better way to communicate. All the information is organized and explained in less than a minute. Furthermore, the resident has a grasp of peripheral issues that significantly characterize the treatment plan, such as the patient's ambulatory status and independence. It is difficult for the attending physician not to appreciate this resident's presentation skills.

NEXT-DAY PREPARATION

Develop a list of patients and their orthopaedic pathologies as you proceed through your nights on call. It is easier to remember facts about problems for which you have personally rendered care. Before your next call day, try to read one article or text selection about each new fracture you have seen. Your knowledge base will grow with little effort. The list of patients will also be useful when you have to pull films for fracture conference or a case presentation.

2

Spinal Column Injuries

GENERAL CONSIDERATIONS AND ASSESSMENT

Stabilization of the Spine

Spinal column injuries deserve special consideration for two main reasons: (1) proper management can, in some situations, prevent permanent paralysis, and (2) these injuries are characteristically severe and have the potential to be life-threatening.

Stabilization of the spine must be achieved from the moment an injured patient is reached by medical personnel. If the spinal column is fractured or dislocated, any movement, even just the head rolling to one side, can twist or impinge on the spinal cord. This may inflict permanent damage or worsen damage that has already occurred. Patients need to be secured onto a "backboard." The backboard looks like a narrow wooden door with cutouts along the sides for hand grips. Some sort of neck stabilization should also be applied, usually a prefabricated collar or neck brace. Sometimes paramedics place sandbags on either side of the head and then place tape across the patient's forehead to keep the head and neck still. In any case, *no manipulation of the neck or back should occur until it is certain that the patient does not have an unstable spinal column injury.*

The backboard itself can become a source of injury because if patients are on it for too long, they can develop skin sores or severe muscle spasm. The backboard can be quickly replaced by an appropriately rigid bed or specialized spinal frame (i.e., a Stryker frame). In fact, no patient should lie on an unpadded backboard for more than a few hours. Transferring patients who are still in the process of a work-up for spinal column injury requires several people to make sure that the patient is moved (or "log-rolled") without twisting or bending the neck or back.

Physical Exam

The physical exam is pivotal in the initial assessment because it establishes the patient's injury as intact, incomplete, or complete. An *intact injury*, of course, is one in which no clinical neurologic deficit is present. An *incomplete injury* is one in which some neurologic deficit is present below a certain level of the spinal cord, but some function below this level also remains. A *complete injury* refers to total loss of neurologic function below a particular level of the spinal cord. Therefore, a injury described as a "C5 complete" would correspond to complete loss of neurologic function below the C5 nerve roots; the level designated in the description corresponds to the lowest completely normal spinal cord level.

Another reason why it is so important to document the physical exam immediately and accurately is because a change in neurologic function has a great impact on treatment. If neurologic function deteriorates, immediate intervention may be warranted, such as emergency surgical decompression of the spinal cord. Improvement of spinal cord function cannot be easily appreciated unless a detailed initial exam is available to serve as a baseline.

The physical exam must be meticulously performed. Knowledge of the body's peripheral nerve organization, dermatome map, and motor reflexes is helpful, because you will be able to more efficiently examine the extremities and torso by testing every motor and sensory level at least once. For example, the upper extremities can be examined by testing biceps power (C5), wrist extension

(C6), finger flexion (C7), and finger adduction (T1). Sensory levels can be examined methodically and quickly by following the dermatome map, and the three critical upper-extremity reflexes are the biceps, triceps, and brachioradialis. Appendix C outlines a simple and thorough exam for spinal cord injury.

Rectal Exam

A rectal exam is of surprising importance in spinal cord assessment for the following reasons:

- It determines the presence of "sacral sparing," an incomplete cord injury in which the sacral levels are intact below a higher injury (thoracic level, for example). Sacral sensibility, however, is limited to a region around the buttocks and anal sphincter, and must be specifically documented.
- Anal sphincter tone is a reflection of sacral level motor function and also must be documented.
- The bulbocavernosus reflex must be recorded (Fig. 2–1). This is a neural reflex that involves a pathway from the genitals to the sacral cord and back to the anal sphincter. Pulling gently on the patient's Foley catheter should elicit some contraction of the anal sphincter. This reflex is important because if it is initially absent and then returns, it signals the end of spinal shock.

The rectal exam, however, always seems to be someone else's job. The neurosurgery service thought you would take care of it, and you thought someone from neurosurgery already did it. As you might expect, it frequently is not initially documented. Do not let this happen on your watch. Do the rectal exam yourself, and do it the first time you examine the patient. Patients with spinal cord injury must have this important feature of the physical exam accurately recorded.

Radiographic Assessment

Standard x-rays are used to "clear" the spine, or establish that it safe to remove the back board and neck brace. For the cervical spine, these are anteroposterior

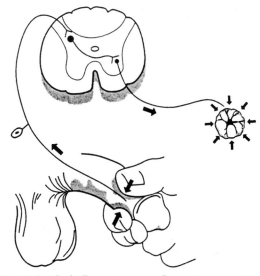

Figure 2–1. The bulbocavernosus reflex arc is a sensorimotor pathway that functions without the use of ascending or descending long tract axons in the spinal cord. When spinal shock resolves, this reflex arc will function even if complete spinal cord disruption is present at a higher level. (From Benson, DR, and Keenan, TL: Evaluation and treatment of trauma to the vertebral column. Instructional Course Lectures, Vol 39. American Academy of Orthopaedic Surgeons, Rosemont, IL, 1990, p 578, with permission.)

(AP), lateral, and open-mouth views, the latter of which is used to see the odontoid in the AP plane. For the thoracolumbar spine, AP and lateral films are sufficient. These films should be obtained in any situation in which spinal injury is suspected and in all situations of multiple trauma.

In some cases, the x-rays may be difficult to assess (e.g., in an uncooperative or severely obese patient), and more sophisticated imaging may be necessary, such as a computed tomography (CT) scan or magnetic resonance imaging (MRI). However, the basic principle of protection must be observed rigorously until the type of injury is clear.

Physiological Effects of Spinal Injury

Patients with spinal cord injury are special because they suffer physiological side effects of central nervous system injury and because they so frequently sustain other very severe injuries. These patients may indeed be among the "sickest" orthopaedic patients with trauma and must be aggressively evaluated. Many hospitals participate in a "Regional Spinal Cord Trauma Center" program in which specific protocols exist for the proper management of such injuries. These centers commonly consult three specialty services as soon as a patient with spinal cord injury is on the way to the ER. These services are orthopaedics, neurosurgery, and respiratory care. General surgery is often involved as well, because abdominal or chest injuries are commonly coexistent. The orthopaedist's role focuses on (1) carefully documenting the neurovascular status of all the extremities and then (2) assessing the imaging studies to identify bony trauma pathology. Be prepared to do your most thorough physical exam, because even subtle weakness or sensory loss may have dramatic implications.

Carefully examine every joint and every bone, because patients frequently cannot communicate clearly or may not be able to feel pain where a fracture is present. You may find that evaluating a patient with spinal cord injury consumes at least 2 hours of your time in the ER, but do not be tempted to cut corners. You cannot leave the patient until you know the full extent of all the injuries. This may mean repeating several x-rays, repeating the physical exam, waiting for other services to complete their initial exam, and then securing proper temporary immobilization or traction as indicated. The initial assessment and management of these patients are time consuming, stressful, and tiring. It is also a team effort, so be professional and supportive in your interactions with other medical staff.

CERVICAL SPINE INJURY: GENERAL PRINCIPLES

The most important relevant history is mechanism of injury and the presence of neck pain. Most cervical spine injuries occur from three mechanisms: a motor vehicle accident, a fall, or a diving accident (i.e., the head hits bottom of pool). In addition to the usual thorough orthopaedic and neurologic assessment, the physical exam should include careful palpation of the neck. Most patients have reproducible tenderness near the specific level of injury. Look for bruising and swelling as well. A very important clue is injury to the forehead or vertex of the skull. Hyperextension injuries that produce cervical fracture often occur by direct impact to the forehead, leaving a forehead bruise or contusion. Similarly, axial load trauma, such as a diving accident, may leave a tell-tale laceration or bump on the skull's vertex. If you know the mechanism, look for corresponding soft-tissue trauma. Conversely, the presence of such associated findings may help you decipher the injury mechanism and also point to more severe underlying pathology.

Radiographic Assessment

The neck must be kept completely immobile until a definitive diagnosis is made. The basic radiographic series includes a lateral view, AP view of the neck, and open-mouth AP views.

Lateral view: The lateral radiograph *must* include all seven cervical vertebrae and the top of T1. It is easy to miss a C7/T1 subluxation because the lateral film did not image below the bottom of C7. Furthermore, obtaining a good lateral x-ray can be difficult because the patient's shoulder routinely blocks visualization of the lower cervical spine. The first way to get a better film is to personally pull down on the patient's arm just at the moment the picture is taken; this will often pull the shoulders down far enough to see the C6 to T1 area. Occasionally in large or obese patients, even pulling down on the arms will represent a challenge and does not improve the lateral film.

The "swimmer's view" is a lateral x-ray taken while one of the patient's arms is forward flexed 180 degrees overhead, as if the patient were swimming freestyle. A lateral x-ray taken in this position does not show the upper cervical spine, but it allows visualization of the lower cervical spine and the first several upper thoracic segments.

AP view: The AP film is helpful to identify disk space narrowing, pedicle abnormalities, and widening of individual vertebral segments.

Open-mouth view: This view is taken with the patient's jaw open so that a clear view of the odontoid process can be obtained. It is essential that this film be included in the basic series, because an odontoid fracture may not be seen with any other view. The lateral film, however, is by far the most valuable of the three because it shows the entire cervical column and highlights any subluxation, fracture, or disk-space narrowing.

Analysis of the Lateral X-ray

Three additional important clues can be obtained from a lateral x-ray:

1. **Prevertebral soft-tissue swelling:** Cervical column injuries reliably produce swelling of the soft tissues immediately anterior to the vertebral bodies. This swelling can easily be measured on a plain lateral x-ray. The normal prevertebral soft-tissue width varies depending on the level, but for the area from C3 to C7, normal width is about 7 to 9 mm. Any significant increase from this size is highly suggestive of significant injury. Look closely and use more sophisticated imaging (e.g., CT scan) if plain films are unclear.
2. **Loss of normal cervical curvature:** The cervical spine normally is slightly lordotic or has a gentle curve that arches forward in its midsection. This curvature is even manifested with the patient lying on a backboard. If the lateral film demonstrates a completely straight cervical spine, this loss of curvature may be the result of pain and muscle spasm. Loss of cervical lordosis should make you suspect that a significant injury is present.
3. **Spinal canal alignment:** A critical feature of any injury is whether or not the spinal cord is encroached. The way to initially assess this is to look

at the borders of the canal as seen on a lateral x-ray. Sometimes the anterior margins of the vertebral bodies will be irregular (even in normal situations) or offset slightly by trauma. The posterior aspect of the body and anterior margin of the spinous process, however, can be seen clearly and should line up to create a continuous smooth contour from one level to the next. If not, the spinal cord is likely to be stretched or compressed.

Additional Imaging Modalities

On occasion, adequate visualization of the cervical spine may not be possible with plain x-rays. Either a good lateral view cannot be obtained, or doubt may remain as to the diagnosis even with good films. In this situation, additional imaging is indicated, usually a CT scan or tomographic series. Sometimes an MRI is also necessary to assess the status of the disk space in the presence of a fracture. Furthermore, the patient's neck must be safely immobilized throughout the work-up. It is not acceptable to remove the patient's neck brace or traction while a CT scan is being obtained. If the brace cannot fit inside the scanner (or if the type of appliance produces too much interference), a physician must hold the patient's neck while the scan is being performed. This is rarely necessary however, because most CT scanners will accommodate braces, and many traction frames now come in graphite compositions to allow a good quality MRI.

Remember that patients with cervical spine injury can decompensate suddenly and often have severe associated injuries. Therefore, do not send these patients to the radiology department alone; you need to go with them and never let them out of your sight. They need to be closely monitored (e.g., pulse oximetry, blood pressure). Many a bad event (critical blood loss, respiratory arrest, etc.) has occurred while the patient was being routed from the x-ray to the CT scanning department. Until the work-up is complete and initial care plan is instituted, these patients must be watched every second.

Immobilization of the Cervical Spine

Traction

If a cervical spinal column fracture or dislocation is clearly present, appropriate immobilization of the neck must be ensured. This means removing the brace or collar, which is a more temporary method of protection, and applying cervical tong traction. Gardner-Wells tongs (Fig. 2–2) are well accepted and available at most centers that receive patients with spinal cord injury. These tongs consist of two sharply pointed pins that are threaded onto a semicircular metal frame. The patient's ears provide the landmarks necessary for tong application.

The tongs should be applied approximately 1 cm superior to the pinna of the ear and about 1 cm posterior to the internal auditory canal opening. This avoids placing

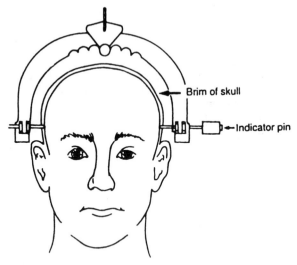

Figure 2–2. Gardner-Wells tongs, used to apply traction and stabilize the cervical spine. (From Frederickson, BE, and Yuan, HA: Nonoperative treatment of the spine: External immobilization. In Browner, BD, Jupiter, JB, Levine, AM, and Trafton, PG [eds]: Skeletal Trauma, 2nd ed. WB Saunders, Philadelphia, 1990, p 815, with permission.)

the tong points near the middle cerebral artery (anterior to the auditory canal) or having the tongs migrate proximally (placed more than 1 cm away form the superior pinna border). Some additional helpful instructions are etched into the metal tong frame.

Usually 5 to 10 lb of weight are added initially, because this amount will offset the weight of the patient's head and apply mild longitudinal pull to the neck. For some fracture patterns, more weight may be appropriate because traction itself can realign the fracture or actually reduce facet dislocations. Although the tongs sound unpleasant, most patients find much better comfort in the stability that they provide.

Specialty Beds

In addition to appropriate traction, the patient should ultimately be transferred to an appropriate bed, such as one of the following:

- The Stryker frame, which allows good access to the patient, incorporates a pulley for cervical traction, and facilitates turning the patient.
- The Rotorest, which is highly adaptable, incorporates traction pulleys and a variety of panel options that allows nursing access and can automatically turn gently from side to side to prevent the development of pressure sores.

Bed and traction preferences may be regional; just remember that formal traction and specialty bed usage need to be implemented soon after the patient with cervical spine injuries is worked up (or if the work-up process takes longer than a few hours).

Treatment Principles

Treatment of cervical spine injuries, like treatment of most spinal disorders, may be highly dependent on surgeon preference and the latest trend in the spine literature. Generally speaking, two basic options exist: closed immobilization or surgery.

Closed immobilization: This is typically accomplished with a halo. This device uses a ring that screws into the skull outer table (much like Gardner-Wells tongs do). Four pins hold the ring to the skull, and vertical metal bars connect the ring to a chest brace that fits over the shoulders and around the upper torso. The halo can be applied at the bedside and is often worn for 6 to 12 weeks or however long it takes the injury to heal. It accomplishes the same degree of immobility achieved with Gardner-Wells tongs but allows the patient to be out of bed and relatively active. Once the decision is made to treat an injury with closed immobilization, patients are typically switched from Gardner-Wells tongs to a halo and mobilized.

Surgery: Surgical management of the cervical spine is often required for two reasons:

1. To remove bony fragments or disk material from the spinal canal to relieve pressure on the spinal cord. This is referred to as "decompression" of the cord. Occasionally this will have to be performed acutely, but many times this is performed semielectively within a day or two of the patient's injury. There is ongoing debate as to whether acute decompression yields more potential for recovery of lost function.
2. To realign fractured or dislocated bony segments that cannot be managed with closed traction. The surgical procedure involves correcting the deformity and then usually fusing an injured segment to a normal adjacent level to effect stability. Fusions can be performed from the posterior aspect of the neck (often secured with wires), or from the front of the neck (often using a fibular strut bone graft and possibly a small metal plate). Sometimes fusions are performed both from the front and back of the neck, depending on the injury severity.

Postoperatively, these patients are commonly protected with a small, removable brace until the fusion heals.

Pediatric Cervical Spine Injury

Children with cervical spine injuries may not demonstrate much or any bony abnormality. This is because ligaments may tear enough to produce instability without necessitating a fracture. A significant mechanism associated with neck pain in a child should be carefully considered as a potential unstable neck injury. This situation has been termed *spinal cord injury without obvious radiographic abnormality (SCIWORA)*. If such injury is suspected, an MRI evaluation is probably warranted.

UPPER CERVICAL SPINE FRACTURES

Fractures of the first two cervical vertebrae can easily be fatal because significant compression of the spinal cord at this level will arrest respiration. With increased attention placed on immobilization of the patient at the scene, aggressive resuscitation, and immediate transport to level 1 trauma centers, more patients with high cervical spine injury are surviving. The most common mechanisms for upper cervical column injury are axial load or hyperextension (or both).

C1 Injury

Clinical Presentation

A *Jefferson's fracture* is fracture of the atlas, or C1 vertebral segment (Fig. 2–3). C1 fractures constitute

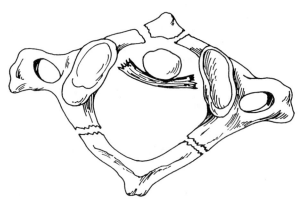

Figure 2–3. Jefferson fracture. (From Errico, TJ, Bauer, RD, and Waugh, T [eds]: Spinal Trauma. JB Lippincott, Philadelphia, 1991, p 147, with permission.)

about 10 percent of cervical spine fractures. The atlas is shaped like a ring and fits over the odontoid process of C2. Visualization of this fracture can be difficult; one clue is widening of the C1 pedicles on the AP view (ring is broken) or break in the ring as seen on a lateral film. The open-mouth view is helpful because the odontoid should be symmetrically surrounded by the "lateral masses" of the atlas. If there is asymmetry or separation between the odontoid and lateral mass of more than 7 mm, an atlas fracture is likely to be the cause. Rotation of the head occurs through the C1-2 junction, so sometimes patients with a C1 fracture will actually present with a malrotated or tilted appearance of their head. Plain films will also show the soft-tissue contour anterior to the atlas, and thickness greater than 10 mm at the anterior arch is strongly suggestive of pathology.

Another way to assess for injury is to obtain flexion and extension lateral x-rays. The distance between the anterior arch of the atlas and the odontoid process should be constant in both positions. The patient must be carefully supervised while obtaining these films so that neurologic injury does not occur.

A common mechanism for the C1 fracture is axial loading, so this fracture is common in diving accidents. Suspect this type of injury when patients present with neck pain and have a bruise or laceration on the vertex of their head.

If plain films do not clearly show the fracture or if a high degree of clinical evidence exists, a CT scan may be the best way to image C1. It is important to know that 50 percent of C1 fractures are associated with other fractures of the cervical spine, and that 25 percent of C1 fractures present with significant cranial and/or facial trauma.

Treatment

Some C1 fractures can be treated with immobilization, and for this purpose, a halo device is used. This effectively immobilizes the neck and head and can be worn for 12 weeks until the cervical fracture has healed. If gross instability is present or decompression of the spinal cord is necessary, sometimes a posterior C1/C2 fusion will be the treatment of choice.

Odontoid Fracture

Odontoid fractures involve the postlike extension of C2 around which the ring of C1 is situated; the odontoid process is also referred to as the *dens*. Odontoid fractures account for about 15 percent of cervical spine fractures. They can result from high-energy neck extension or flexion mechanisms as well as from relatively minor falls. Patients have been known to report a strange feeling "as if my head were going to fall off unless I hold it."

Odontoid fractures are very easy to miss. The open-mouth view may sometimes be the only x-ray that shows the fracture; a CT scan may be required to show adequate detail. Furthermore, odontoid fractures in children can be very difficult to assess because the odontoid process normally has four ossification centers, all of which appear like fractures in the skeletally immature patient. An MRI can be very helpful in looking for hematoma and other soft-tissue findings associated with a fracture.

There are three types of odontoid fractures (classified by Anderson and D'Alonzo) (Fig. 2–4).

- *Type I fracture* occurs at its distal tip and typically heals with closed immobilization.
- *Type II fracture* occurs through the shaft of the odontoid process. Nonunion of this type is relatively common and seems to be more likely when initial displacement is greater than 6 mm, the patient is older than 60 years, and displacement is posteriorly directed. Surgical management of the type II fracture (usually posterior C1/C2 fusion) is indicated if nonunion seems to be likely; however, the decision to proceed with operative care instead of halo immobilization may be a difficult one in very elderly patients.
- *Type III fracture* occurs at the base of the odontoid where it attaches to the body of C2; this variant is often treated with a halo.

C2 Pedicle Fracture

Another common fracture of C2 (or *axis*) is through the bony posterior elements (Fig. 2–5). Fracture

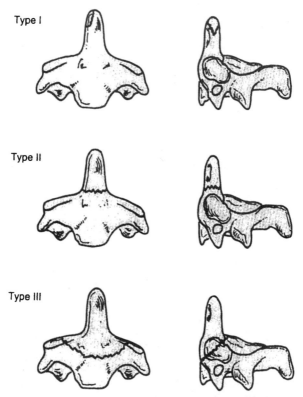

Type I

Type II

Type III

Figure 2–4. The Anderson and D'Alonzo classification of odontoid fractures. Type I fractures occur at the tip; type II fractures involve the odontoid base; type III fractures extend into the C2 body. (From Frederickson, BE, and Yuan, HA: Nonoperative treatment of the spine: External immobilization. In Browner, BD, Jupiter, JB, Levine, AM, and Trafton, PG [eds]: Skeletal Trauma, 2nd ed. WB Saunders, Philadelphia, 1990, p 820, with permission.)

through the pedicle of C2 has been called the *hangman's fracture* because it was produced by extension and distraction characterizing judicial hanging. Nowadays it is the extension and axial load of motor vehicle accidents that produce the most common C2 posterior element injuries.

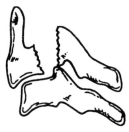

Figure 2–5. A C2 pedicle fracture, also called the "hangman's fracture." (From Frederickson, BE, and Yuan, HA: Nonoperative treatment of the spine: External immobilization. In Browner, BD, Jupiter, JB, Levine, AM, and Trafton, PG [eds]: Skeletal Trauma, 2nd ed. WB Saunders, Philadelphia, 1990, p 821, with permission.)

Treatment

The following are treatment options for C2 pedicle fractures:

- **Brace immobilization:** usually the treatment of choice for an injury that has not produced displacement of more than 3 mm
- **Traction:** used to improve position if more displacement or instability is present; then halo immobilization is typically recommended until healing occurs (12 weeks)
- **Surgical intervention:** used in rare cases of severe deformity and instability

LOWER CERVICAL SPINE INJURIES

The most common injury patterns between C3 and C7 are facet dissociation, vertebral body fracture, and extension injuries. Central to the management of these fractures is whether or not instability exists. Instability means that enough of the bony and ligamentous support elements have been disrupted to allow unphysiological motion at one or more vertebral segments, which among other things, will threaten the spinal cord. A variety of criteria have been established to characterize instability. Two important radiographic findings are vertebral body translation of more than 3.5 mm or angulation between two segments of more than 11 degrees.

Facet Dislocation

Facet dislocations present in two main varieties (Fig. 2–6):

1. A *unilateral facet dislocation* represents the dislocation of an inferior facet anterior to the superior one. On lateral film, the inferior vertebral body will appear to be subluxed about 25 percent forward. An oblique film better demonstrates the dislocation.
2. *Bilateral facet dislocation* ("jumped" facets) produces a subluxation of 50 percent or more on lateral film.

Facet dislocation, especially the bilateral type, can produce significant cord compression and neurologic injury.

Closed reduction can often be accomplished by application of traction, although bilateral facet reduction may require manipulation under anesthesia. Any manipulation performed must be done with extreme care so as to not worsen any cord compromise. Evidence suggests that immediate relief of pressure on the spinal cord can prevent some degree of permanent injury. Facet dislocations represent primarily ligamentous injury. Consequently, stability must usually be restored through surgical fusion, commonly through a posterior approach.

Vertebral Body Fracture

Vertebral body fractures come in three main types:

1. *Compression fractures* result from flexion and compression forces and are measured according to the amount of vertebral body height lost. If the injury represents less than 25 percent of lost height, symptomatic care and use of a brace is appropriate. When more than 50 percent of the body is compressed, the posterior ligamentous structures can be torn and treatment commonly includes operative stabilization (sometimes an anterior and posterior ap-

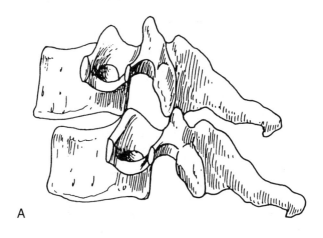

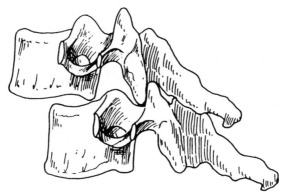

Figure 2–6. (*A*) A 25 percent forward displacement of the upper vertebral segment suggests a unilateral facet dislocation. (*B*) Anterior displacement of 50 percent or more is consistent with a bilateral facet dislocation. (From Errico, TJ, Bauer, RD, and Waugh, T [eds]: Spinal Trauma. JB Lippincott, Philadelphia, 1991, p 152, with permission)

proach). Furthermore, there is a greater risk of cord compression due to bony fragment impingement or disk extrusion.

2. *Vertebral body burst fractures* are the result of more pure compression, without a flexion vector. Fracture

pieces are frequently extruded backwards into the spinal canal. Stabilization requires anterior vertebrectomy and fusion, with or without plate fixation.
3. *Teardrop fracture-dislocations* are so called because the triangular piece of bone is broken off the anterior inferior edge of the lower vertebral body. The involved level is often displaced posteriorly, highlighting the high-energy nature of this injury. Because of gross instability, these injuries require at least an anterior fusion; some authors also recommend posterior wiring.

Extension trauma results from compression of the neck in an extended posture (see Fig. 2-5). A teardrop fracture can occur, but in this case, it is an avulsion fracture. Frequently, posterior bony elements, such as the lamina, are crushed. If significant instability results, a posterior fusion is mandated. Less severe extension injuries (without gross instability or cord encroachment) can be treated with a brace.

Spinous Process Avulsion

The "clay shoveler's" fracture is an avulsion fracture of the C7 spinous process. This occurs from sudden, extreme muscle contraction. Supervised flexion and extension lateral x-rays can be obtained to make sure no instability exists. Then symptomatic care is sufficient until the fracture heals.

THORACOLUMBAR INJURIES

Fractures of the thoracic and lumbar spine can be classified into four types: wedge compression, burst, flexion-distraction, and translational. As in the cervical spine, a key determinant of treatment and outcome relates to the fracture's inherent stability. Unstable fractures are more likely the result of high-energy trauma and are more likely to require operative management to restore alignment and stability.

Denis has described a three-column model for the spine based on anatomic landmarks. Unstable fractures typically involve damage to two or more of these columns.

1. The anterior column is the anterior longitudinal ligament and the anterior half of the vertebral body and disk material.
2. The middle column is the posterior longitudinal ligament and the posterior half of the vertebral body and disk.
3. The posterior column consists of the bony arch and posterior ligamentous structures.

Radiographic assessment depends on good AP and lateral films. It is also important to ask the radiology technician to shoot an extra lateral film centered about the lumbosacral junction. This film is key to assessing the lower lumbar spine and sacrum.

Compression Fracture

Wedge compression fractures (Fig. 2–7) result from sudden flexion of the back. As in the cervical spine, loss of vertebral body height of more than 50 percent means that some posterior damage is present. This increases the likelihood of spinal cord compromise and need for surgical intervention. Minimal (<25 percent) compression fractures are very common in osteopenic patients. These fractures often occur without any history of trauma and are treated symptomatically. Be careful, however, to meticulously screen the films for metastatic disease (that may have caused the vertebral body to collapse). Also, be aware that sudden significant collapse of the vertebral body, even in an elderly osteopenic patient, can produce spinal canal encroachment.

Burst Fracture

Burst fractures are caused by longitudinal load and occur most frequently at the L1 level. This is because the thoracolumbar junction is the junction of two large motion segments (thoracic spine and lumbar spine). An AP view is useful because it will demonstrate widening of the pedicle at the involved level. Retropulsion of bony fragments can narrow the spinal canal or actually impinge the cord directly. This then requires decompression (usually through an anterior approach) and fusion (anterior and possibly posterior).

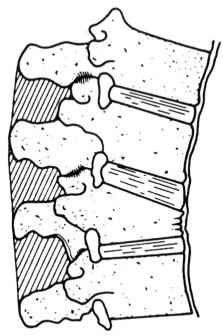

Figure 2–7. An example of a wedge compression-type fracture of the lumbar spine. (From Mueller, FO, and Ryan, AJ: Prevention of Athletic Injuries: The Role of the Sports Medicine Team. FA Davis, Philadelphia, 1991, p. 204, with permission.)

Flexion-Distraction Injury

Flexion-distraction injuries start with a flexion moment anterior to the spine. Then, in the injury process, a distraction or stretching type force results in further displacement of the injured parts (see Fig. 2-6). A stable example of this injury type is the *Chance fracture*, which has been associated with sudden deceleration in a seat-belted passenger. This produces a transverse fracture through all three columns, but the anterior longitudinal ligament is preserved and there's no anterior column displacement. Because this is a stable pattern, Chance fractures can often be managed with brace immobilization.

Translational Injury

Translational injuries result from a combination of forces and typically involve severe disruption of all three columns. Consequently, these injuries are highly unstable and almost always result in severe spinal cord injury. The gross instability and malalignment of the spinal column elements mandate surgical stabilization.

SACRAL INJURIES

Fractures of the sacrum do not have the same potential for spinal cord injury as fractures of the upper spinal column because the spinal cord proper has ended proximally. However, sacral fractures can be associated with high-energy trauma. Therefore, patients must be carefully screened. Furthermore, fractures that involve the sacra foramina can indeed compromise the associated nerve root or the nearby lumbosacral nerve plexus. It is also important to note sacral fractures that involve the sacroiliac joint, because significant deformity can produce painful arthritis. Sacroiliac disruption may also represent the posterior component of an unstable pelvic fracture, so be certain to carefully evaluate (physical exam and x-ray) the entire pelvic ring.

The coccyx is the most distal tip of the sacrum and injury to this area can result from a fall directly onto the buttocks. It can be difficult to specifically identify a fracture here, even with a good lateral sacral film. However, even if a displaced coccygeal fracture is present, treatment consists of symptomatic care until the fracture heals. Warn patients that injuries to the coccyx can be intermittently sore for many months before they finally resolve.

3
CHAPTER

Pelvic Fractures

GENERAL CONSIDERATIONS

Fractures of the pelvis deserve respect because, like spinal column injuries, they can be rapidly fatal. Furthermore, although most pelvic fractures are stable and nonsurgically treated, the difference between a simple injury pattern and a serious one may not be immediately obvious to the inexperienced.

Initial Assessment

The initial assessment of pelvic fractures is similar to that for multiple-trauma injuries (see Chap. 1). Pelvic fractures can represent high-energy injuries, and an estimated 60 to 85 percent of these patients have fractures in other extremities. Closed head injury, abdominal injury, and pulmonary trauma also closely correlate with the presence of pelvic fracture.

Physical Exam

As in any patient with potential multiple-trauma injury, the physical exam should include a thorough assessment of the spinal column and all extremities. The physical exam of the pelvis itself is also important. The following is the suggested protocol for the pelvic exam:

1. Palpate the bony prominences, including the iliac crests (anterior and posterior), the pubic rami and symphysis, and the ischial tuberosities.
2. Note any tenderness or bony instability. Peculiar positioning of a lower extremity, either in internal or external rotation, will also be a clue to distortion of pelvic anatomy.
3. Neurologic examination of the lower extremities is relevant because 50 percent of unstable pelvic fractures produce injury to the lumbosacral plexus.
4. Rectal and vaginal exams are essential because pelvic fractures have the potential to tear through these areas, becoming open fractures. Swelling and bruising of the scrotum or labia suggest pelvic hematoma. Carefully note whether there is any blood at the urethral opening, which would suggest bladder and/or urethral injury. The perineum tends to be an area that many examiners avoid; do not make this mistake. In the same way that patients with multiple trauma must be completely undressed and searched for all possible injuries, patients with pelvic fracture must have their perineum examined carefully. A missed vaginal laceration or open colon perforation from a pelvic fracture has been associated with a 50 percent mortality rate.

Pelvic Fracture and Hypotension

In concert with the physical exam, the patient's vital signs must be assessed and monitored closely. Retroperitoneal hemorrhage causes 60 percent of deaths in patients with pelvic fractures. A mortality rate of 38 percent has been attributed to patients who present in a hypotensive state compared with only 3 percent in those with normal blood pressure at admission. This fact underscores the need for immediate aggressive resuscitation.

Although major pelvic fractures can easily produce hypotension, patients frequently sustain other injuries that can produce abnormal hemodynamics. Therefore, do not assume that the pelvis is the main or only source of bleeding. Other possible sources are the thoracic cavity and abdominal cavity in addition to the retroperitoneal space.

The general surgery service is usually trauma team leader and will pursue assessment of bleeding in the abdominal and thoracic areas. However, the orthopaedic surgeon is an integral part of the pelvic fracture management process, and you should know the general protocol for evaluating patients with these complicated injuries.

The following are key points in managing the patient with pelvic fracture and hypotension:

1. Fluid resuscitation is begun immediately (via multiple large-bore IV sites). Next, the trauma service will likely pursue ultrasound, computed tomography (CT) scan, or diagnostic peritoneal lavage (DPL) to determine the presence of abdominal bleeding.
2. If the DPL is positive (10 to 20 mL of blood aspirated), exploratory laparotomy is emergently performed by the trauma service. It is important for the orthopaedic team to be present at this procedure because some element of definitive management for the pelvic fracture may relate to the procedure. For example, it may help to apply an external fixator in the operating room just before the laparotomy to stabilize the pelvis or reduce bleeding.
3. The temporary fixation may be modified at the conclusion of the laparotomy.
4. Alternatively, the laparotomy incision might be extended, allowing definitive plate fixation of an anteriorly unstable fracture.

Whatever the exact details, the orthopaedic surgeon must maintain direct participation while the patient is in the operating room, because some treatment decisions can be made more efficiently if the general surgery and orthopaedic surgery services work together.

Management of Hemorrhage

The following have been identified as the most common sources of bleeding in patients with pelvic fracture:

- Exposed cancellous bone surfaces at the fracture site
- Retroperitoneal lumbar venous disruption
- Local arterial injury

It is interesting that arterial injury accounts for only 20 percent of major bleeding cases (most common vessel: internal pudendal artery), and that most of the blood loss occurs from a low pressure source.

If the DPL is negative and the pelvis seems to be the most likely source of hypotension (i.e., unstable fracture pattern), additional intervention must proceed to characterize and control retroperitoneal hematoma. Angiography may be used to identify the active bleeding source as well as to effect embolization to arrest hemorrhage. Furthermore, external fixation can be applied emergently; this can stabilize the pelvis anteriorly, reduce the overall pelvic volume, and facilitate retroperitoneal tamponade.

Urinary Tract Injury

Placement of a Foley catheter is important in a patient with pelvic fracture because close monitoring of fluid status is required. Although the catheter does not need to be placed in the first few minutes of admission, patients with major trauma typically have a catheter placed during their initial work-up in the emergency room (ER). *Completely blind placement of a Foley catheter can impart serious additional trauma if the urethra and/or bladder are injured.* Therefore, many clinicians recommend performing a retrograde urethrogram and cystogram first. This involves placing a small amount of contrast medium into the urethra and bladder and then obtaining an x-ray. If a urethral laceration or bladder rupture is present, extravasation of dye will identify the problem. Remember that upon physical exam, blood at the urethral opening is highly suggestive of urinary tract damage.

In male patients, the rectal exam can identify not only blood or mucosal tears, but also abnormal position of the prostate, which is also suggestive of urethral injury. If the retrograde urethrogram is normal, then a Foley catheter can be placed more confidently. However, extreme care should be exercised even if the urethrogram is normal. Never force catheter placement of the Foley or proceed if extreme pain occurs.

In urethral injury, the urology service typically will place a suprapubic catheter. In this way, urine can be drained without using or manipulating injured passageways. Similarly, patients with rectal or colonic injuries commonly undergo placement of a colostomy. The colostomy diverts waste material away from the fracture site and lacerated soft tissues and is key in preventing patients with open pelvic fractures from becoming septic. *Missed open pelvic fractures have a 50 percent mortality rate, and sepsis is a primary cause of death.*

Deep Venous Thrombosis

Patients with pelvic fracture are at extremely high risk for developing deep venous thrombosis. The rate of pulmonary embolism in this population has been reported to be as high as 2 percent, compared with only 0.2 percent in patients with multiple trauma without pelvic fracture. Therefore, after hemorrhage has been controlled, patients should be given anticoagulants. In those patients for whom anticoagulant medication is contraindicated, a vena caval filter may be placed.

Radiographic Assessment

Radiographic evaluation starts with a simple AP film. Once the initial trauma assessment and resuscitation process are under way, several additional films, called "Judet views," can be very helpful:

1. An obturator oblique film is taken with the injured side turned 45 degrees toward the x-ray beam and highlights the anterior pelvic column and posterior wall of the acetabulum (Fig. 3–1).
2. The iliac oblique film is obtained with the injured side turned 45 degrees away from the x-ray beam and highlights the posterior pelvic column and anterior acetabular wall (Fig. 3–2).

Inlet and outlet views are AP films taken with the x-ray beam angled 45 degrees caudad and cephalad. These films highlight anatomy of the pubic rami and sacroiliac joints. Also, note that for almost every pelvic fracture other than simple rami fractures, a CT scan should be obtained, because this modality yields a greater amount of detail that plain x-ray may not depict.

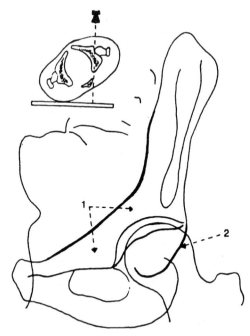

Figure 3–1. The obturator oblique view of the pelvis. This view highlights the anterior border of the iliac wing (1), and the posterior lip of the acetabulum (2). (From Judet, R, Judet, J, and Letournel, E: Fractures of the acetabulum: Classification and surgical approaches for open reduction. Preliminary report. J Bone Joint Surg 46A:1617, 1964, with permission.)

Sometimes, a CT scan is ordered by the general surgery service to assess the abdominal contents. Ask the technician to continue the imaging sequence through the pelvis and you will have saved the patient a trip back to the scanner.

Postinjury Mobilization

Early mobilization of patients with pelvic fractures, like most patients with multiple trauma, correlates with a faster and less complicated recovery. This is probably related to a lower incidence of pulmonary and throm-

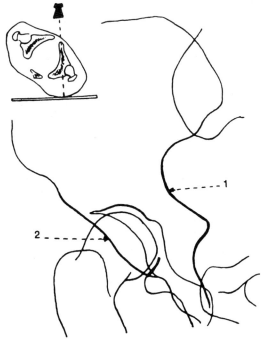

Figure 3–2. The iliac oblique view of the pelvis. This view highlights (1) the posterior wall of the iliac bone and (2) the anterior margin of the acetabulum. (From Judet, R, Judet, J, and Letournel, E: Fractures of the acetabulum: Classification and surgical approaches for open reduction. Preliminary report. J Bone Joint Surg 46A:1617, 1964, with permission.)

botic complications. After initial resuscitation, definitive management typically focuses not only on restoration of anatomy but also on enabling ambulation as soon as possible.

SPECIFIC INJURIES

Complex Pelvic Ring Injury

The pelvis can be thought of as a ring consisting of the iliac wings, connected anteriorly through the pubic rami and symphysis pubis, and connected posteriorly through the sacrum. Minor injury involves disruption of only one part of the ring, whereas more significant trauma will cause the ring to be disrupted in several locations, allowing part of the ring to shift entirely.

Classification

Pelvic ring injuries have been classified by Young and Burgess based on mechanism of injury to the ring. The main categories are lateral compression, anteroposterior compression, and vertical shear (sometimes called the *Malgaigne fracture;* Fig. 3–3 A, B, and C). Each category can be divided into several grades, based on amount of ring disruption. A fourth category has also been described that takes into account combined mechanisms (anterolateral force and anterovertical force). See Figure 3–3 for some examples of unstable pelvic fracture patterns.

Treatment Principles

The following are management principles for pelvic ring injuries:

1. *Restoration of stability to an unstable ring* is an important principle of treatment. If the ring is broken in two locations, a segment of the pelvis will be mobile. For example, with a type II vertical shear fracture, part of the iliac wing and included acetabulum can shift superiorly with respect to the rest of the pelvis. Treatment focuses on realigning the shifted segment and then conferring stability through internal fixation (i.e., plating the iliac wing and the rami fractures).

2. *External fixation* is one method of conferring stability to the anterior pelvis. It may be also attractive because of its use in controlling severe hemorrhage in the acute injury period. Posterior stability (iliac wing fracture and sacroiliac joint disruption) is commonly achieved with screws and plates.

3. *Surgical intervention* for pelvic ring injuries is commonly pursued within 5 to 7 days of presentation. Many surgeons prefer to wait this period to stabilize the patient's physiology, carefully assess and plan

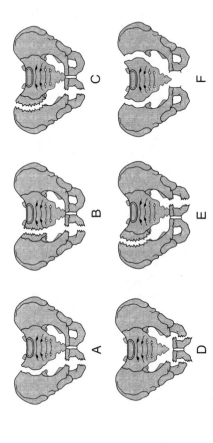

Figure 3–3. Examples of unstable pelvic fractures. (*A*), (*B*), and (*C*) illustrate vertical shear (Malgaigne) types, involving the ischiopubic rami and disruption of an ipsilateral sacroiliac joint. (*D*) is an example of a straddle fracture involving all four pubic rami. (*E*) shows a bucket handle fracture involving an ischiopubic ramus and a contralateral sacroiliac joint. (*F*) shows disruption of both sacroiliac joints and the pubic symphysis. (From McKinnis, LN: Fundamentals of Orthopedic Radiology. FA Davis, Philadelphia, 1997, p 225, with permission.)

treatment of other injuries, and perhaps most important, allow potentially massive retroperitoneal hematoma to reach equilibrium.

Symphysis Pubis Injury

Disruptions of the symphysis may represent the anterior break of the pelvic ring or they may be isolated injuries. Be sure to assess the other parts of the pelvic ring for disruptions that could characterize an unstable situation.

For isolated symphysis separations, nonsurgical care is appropriate if the separation is less than 2.5 cm. Diastasis greater than this is often treated with plate fixation, except in the case of symphysis separation due to childbirth. Even dramatic diastasis in the new mother can often be just followed up symptomatically because, in most of these cases, the separation closes down by itself and becomes asymptomatic and stable.

Pubic Ramus Fracture

Fractures of the pubic ramus are extremely common as isolated entities, especially in the elderly. A low-energy fall is often the cause. Make sure no posterior disruption is present, such as widening of the sacroiliac joint, which might characterize the injury as more severe. Straddle fractures, or bilateral rami fractures, can be associated with posterior ring instability and can be grossly unstable. The history and physical exam typically guide you to the proper scenario. For example, a 90-year-old who fell out of a chair at home is likely to have an injury personality quite different from that of a 35-year-old equestrian who was thrown into a fence.

Although the isolated pubic ramus fracture can be very painful, by itself it does not compromise the weight-bearing axis of the pelvis. Therefore, immediate ambulation is possible and to be encouraged. However, because this fracture commonly occurs in elderly, partially compromised patients, admission to the hospital often results. The patients may require narcotic pain medication for 1 or 2 days and almost always benefit from the supervision of a physical therapist. Do not overmedicate. Elderly individuals may be acutely sensitive to small doses of narcotics. Resumption of ambulation (often with a walker) can be accomplished within a few days as discomfort improves, and then the patient is discharged.

Iliac Wing Fracture

Iliac wing fractures are amenable to plate fixation because of the available flat bony surfaces. Indications

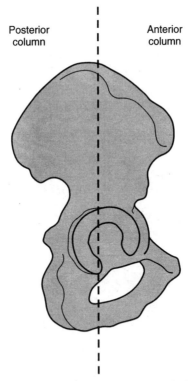

Posterior column

Anterior column

Figure 3–4. The innominate bone and acetabulum can be divided into anterior and posterior columns. (From McKinnis, LN: Fundamentals of Orthopedic Radiology. FA Davis, Philadelphia, 1997, p 227, with permission.)

for fixation depend on what other disruption is present in the pelvic ring. Iliac fractures typically occur from high-energy trauma, and open wounds can significantly complicate the management of patients with these fractures.

Sacroiliac Disruption

Injury is significant because the sacroiliac (SI) joint represents a major posterior junction in the pelvic ring. Furthermore, the ligaments around this joint are among the biggest and strongest in the body. Widening of the SI joint, therefore, deserves respect. If there is an anterior disruption of the pelvis, some form of stabilization must be effected, often anteriorly and posteriorly. Large lag screws are often the method of fixation for the SI joint. Sacral fracture may also require operative attention if a sacral nerve root is compromised or if there is significant incongruity of the SI joint articular surfaces.

Acetabular Fracture

The anatomy of acetabular fracture is difficult to understand because the shape of the bone is so complex. Letournel's classification is the most commonly used

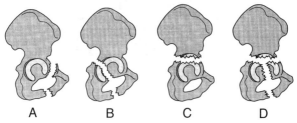

Figure 3–5. Examples of acetabular fractures: (*A*) anterior column; (*B*) posterior column; (*C*) transverse, involving both columns; (*D*) complex or T-shaped, which also involves both columns. (From McKinnis, LN: Fundamentals of Orthopedic Radiology. FA Davis, Philadelphia, 1997, p 227, with permission.)

and depends on organizing the acetabulum into zones called columns and walls (Fig. 3–4). The fracture is then also further categorized as being anterior, posterior, or both (transverse) (Fig. 3–5). Specific treatment, such as style of internal fixation and operative exposure, depends on the exact fracture anatomy. You should be aware that most acetabular fractures with any significant displacement require operative care. Even minor changes in the acetabular congruity can produce devastating long-term effects on the hip joint, because this joint is so heavily and frequently loaded. Even the most aggressive surgical intervention for certain severe fractures may not be able to prevent development of post-traumatic arthritis years after the injury.

4

Adult Upper-Extremity Fractures

This chapter covers 13 major types of upper-extremity fractures. As is true for most of this book, it is written to answer the resident's questions while in the emergency room (ER). In particular, "What do I need to know *right now* to begin treating a patient in the ER with one of these injuries?" Fracture classification is reviewed briefly, focusing on the common and simplest classification schemes. Definitive fracture care is also noted in most cases so that the resident will understand possible requirements for the patient's total care. In this way, the patient's general expectations for care can be properly guided right from the first contact with the orthopaedic service in the ER. The resident can later check complete information about each condition in a major textbook when more time is available. Remember, the following fracture care is just an introduction to help you when first evaluating patients. It is *not* a substitute for thorough review of a definitive text.

CLAVICULAR FRACTURES

Clinical Assessment

Fracture of the clavicle is very common and occurs typically from a moderate fall (from a bicycle or down a few stairs) or from blows during a contact sport. Patients complain of sharp shoulder pain and are reluctant to move the upper extremity on the injured side. Verify that no neck pain or upper-extremity paresthesias are present.

Physical exam will confirm sharp tenderness at the fracture site, which will appear swollen and crepitant. Gentle, controlled passive motion of the shoulder is usually possible with minimal discomfort. Clavicle fractures can also be associated with high-energy trauma (motor vehicle accidents) and may, in those cases, be accompanied by the following, more ominous, associated injuries:

First rib fracture
Scapular fracture
Open clavicle fracture
Subclavian vein thrombosis
Pneumothorax
Brachial plexus injury
Cervical spine injury

Be sure to screen for these less common, but serious, problems in both history and physical exam.

Radiographic Evaluation

Primary radiographic evaluation consists of an AP clavicle view and a 30-degree cephalad view, the latter of which will isolate the clavicle from the first rib. Very distal clavicle fractures may justify an axial view or additional views to characterize the shoulder.

Classification is according to location in the proximal, middle, or distal third. Neer has subclassified distal third fractures according to location relative to the coracoclavicular (CC) and acromioclavicular (AC) ligaments:

- Distal third type I—between the CC and AC ligaments
- Distal third type II—medial to CC ligaments
- Distal third type III—at AC joint

Treatment Considerations

Clavicle fractures very rarely require any operative intervention. Even comminuted or dramatically displaced fractures usually heal spontaneously. Symptomatic nonunions can occur but are rare.

Initial treatment for isolated clavicular fractures consists of immobilizing the upper extremity on the injured side. This can be accomplished with a simple sling or a shoulder immobilizer. A "figure-of-eight" harness is another device that may also be helpful because it can pull the shoulder posteriorly and reduce pain and immediate deformity. This harness, however, does not significantly affect alignment of the healed fracture; in fact, all appliances are merely for comfort and protection during the healing period. If a figure-of-eight strap is used, it should be removed if any skin irritation or direct pressure occurs over the fracture site.

Patients should be told that the injury may be quite painful and palpably unstable for up to 1 month, and that solid union may require 8 to 10 weeks. A permanent deformity presenting as a "bump" at the fracture site is inevitable and may be very noticeable in patients with little subcutaneous fat over the bone. Oftentimes the education and instruction that patients require for this fracture are inversely proportional to the amount of actual intervention needed beyond use of a sling. Type II distal third clavicle fractures can produce a marked deformity. Type I and type III distal third clavicle fractures are more stable, because the coracoclavicular (CC) ligaments are still connected to the medial (shaft) portion of the fracture. The type II injury, however, occurs such that the fracture functionally detaches the clavicle shaft from the CC ligaments, and the shaft then tends to elevate dramatically. The deformity as well as the greater potential for nonunion are concerns in this situation. Consequently, some surgeons prefer to treat type II distal third clavicle fractures with acute operative stabilization, either by pinning the fracture or tying the clavicle shaft down to the coracoid process with heavy suture. Nonetheless, even for the type II injury, nonoperative treatment often produces an excellent functional result (albeit with a bump at the injury site) and many orthopaedists reserve operative intervention only if

closed management fails to yield a painless, strong
shoulder.

SCAPULAR FRACTURES (INCLUDING THE GLENOID)

Clinical Assessment

Scapular fractures are relatively rare, and high-
energy trauma is typically involved. Also, associated
injuries are common. Include in the physical examination assessment of the neck and ribs as well as the
neurovascular status of the involved extremity. Radiographic evaluation should include an AP of the shoulder, a scapular "Y" view, an axillary view, and a chest
x-ray. Classification is based on the part of the scapula
primarily involved:

- Type I—body of the scapula
- Type II—coracoid and acromion
- Type III—neck and glenoid

Ideberg has further classified glenoid fractures into
five types, depending on the location and complexity
of the fracture (Fig. 4–1). A computed tomography (CT)
scan can be helpful in identifying the exact geometry
of the injury.

Treatment Considerations

Treatment for most scapular fractures is nonoperative. Initial management of the fracture may involve just
placing the arm in a sling to reduce shoulder motion. If
the patient has not had multiple trauma and is able to
go home from the ER, careful early follow-up should
be planned so that appropriate imaging studies can be
obtained and definitive fracture management planned.
Surgical intervention may be necessary if any of the
following are present:

- Certain types of glenoid fractures in which large
  fragments are displaced (>25% of joint surface)
- Significant articular incongruity (>2 mm)
- Humeral head subluxation

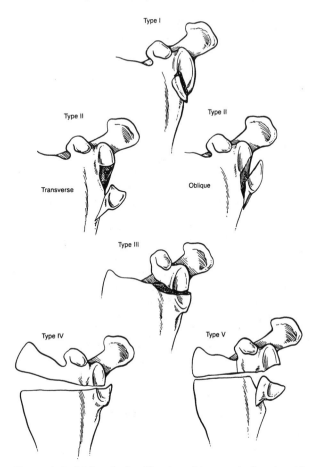

Figure 4–1. Ideberg's classification of intra-articular glenoid fractures. (From Rockwood, CA, Jr., and Matsen, FA, III [eds]: The Shoulder. WB Saunders, Philadelphia, 1990, p 348, with permission.)

Key features in managing these patients may be identifying and treating associated trauma to the neck, shoulder, or chest (e.g., cervical spine fracture, first rib fracture, flail chest, brachial plexus injury). Scapular and first rib fractures have a high correlation with pulmonary and neurovascular injuries.

PROXIMAL HUMERAL FRACTURES

Clinical Assessment

Particularly common in the elderly, proximal humeral fractures are frequently sustained from low-energy trauma. In addition to neck and elbow pain, the presence of paresthesias is an important aspect of the history, because brachial plexus stretch injuries may be present, and occasionally axillary artery injury accompanies this fracture in older patients with calcified vessels.

In younger patients, the energy of trauma is typically higher, so be certain to assess adjacent areas for injury.

Physical examination is marked by the following:

- Tenderness and crepitance at the proximal arm
- Frequent development of dramatic ecchymosis, spreading to the anterior chest and distally to the forearm during the first week after injury

Shoulder range of motion is not particularly helpful in assessment because such activity produces movement at the fracture site rather than the glenohumeral joint. Carefully check and document the upper-extremity neurovascular status, including distal pulses. Palpate about the shoulder to help detect an accompanying dislocation of the humeral head.

Radiographic Evaluation

Radiographic evaluation must include at least two orthogonal views: an AP view of the shoulder (or even better, a true AP of the glenoid) and either an axillary lateral or a scapular Y lateral view. The advantage of the latter view is that the patient's arm does not have to be abducted or held uncomfortably. Radiographic evaluation should not only demonstrate the fracture pattern, but also confirm that a dislocation, particularly a posterior dislocation (commonly missed), is not present. Although not often ordered in the ER, a CT scan of the shoulder can be useful for planning definitive treatment of complex fracture patterns.

Neer has classified displaced proximal humeral fractures based on the number of fracture "parts." A bony fragment qualifies as a "part" if it is displaced more than 1 cm or angulated more than 45 degrees.

Treatment Considerations

Unless vascular compromise, glenohumeral dislocation, or an open fracture is present, proximal humeral fractures can be treated initially in the ER with a sling or shoulder immobilizer. Emphasize early office follow-up for further evaluation and definitive care. Occasionally, manipulation of the arm produces better alignment of the fracture pieces, although only one or two attempts at manipulation are recommended.

Approximately 85 percent of these fractures do not require any operative management. Some two-part fractures will be completely displaced, with the humeral shaft being pulled anterior and medial by muscle attachments. When there is complete displacement or no bony contact between the parts, often a closed reduction and pinning (or even open reduction) may be required. Patients with significantly displaced three-part fractures may be candidates for a formal open reduction with internal fixation, and patients with most badly displaced four-part fractures require a humeral hemiarthroplasty.

Remember that most proximal humerus fractures are impacted and partially stable and consequently require only a sling for comfort and physical therapy as soon as partial healing allows (2 to 4 weeks). Key features of decision making include relative displacement of the fragments and glenohumeral articular congruity.

Isolated fractures of the tuberosities can occur, and the greater tuberosity fracture is most common. If significantly displaced (same Neer criteria), then ORIF is usually recommended. ER care consists of sling immobilization and early follow-up in the office to plan definitive care.

Associated Dislocations

Humeral head splitting fractures do particularly poorly, and most require hemiarthroplasty (on a semi-elective basis) if the involved segment is greater than

45 percent of the humeral head. Associated dislocation of the glenohumeral joint also reflects a greater degree of injury than an isolated proximal humeral fracture. Immediate care mandates that the dislocation be reduced. It is therefore critical that the ER evaluation identify when a dislocation is present.

HUMERAL SHAFT FRACTURES

Clinical Assessment

Humeral shaft fractures can be caused by a direct blow or a twisting movement, which will produce a spiral or oblique fracture line. Gross instability of the arm and sharp pain usually account for patients holding the injured extremity apprehensively.

Physical exam should include a careful exam of the extremity's neurovascular status. Distal third humeral shaft fractures (Holstein-Lewis) are associated with radial nerve injury (Fig. 4–2).

Radiographic evaluation consists of AP and lateral views of the entire humerus (shoulder to elbow). The best lateral view is a "shoot-through"; the x-ray machine (not the arm) must be moved to obtain this view, and usually an assistant must hold the extremity. Classification of humeral shaft fractures relates primarily to location (proximal, middle, or distal third) and to fracture pattern (e.g., transverse, oblique, spiral).

Initial Treatment

Immediate care consists of splinting the extremity by means of one of the following techniques: a hanging cast, a coaptation splint ("sugar tong"), and a "collar and cuff."

Reduction of the fracture may occur just with gentle gravity traction. Use of a regular arm sling tends to support the elbow and often pulls the distal shaft segment superiorly, producing angulation or displacement. A collar and cuff is basically a strap that goes around the patient's neck (collar) and then wraps around the wrist (cuff). This device holds the forearm parallel with the floor and supports the arm but does

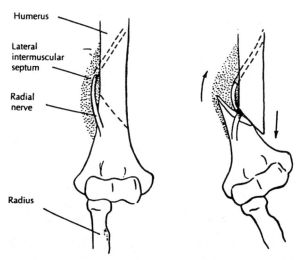

Figure 4–2. Distal third humeral fracture (Holstein-Lewis type). Note potential for the radial nerve to become entrapped in the fracture site. (From Holstein, A, and Lewis, GB: Fractures of the humerus with radial nerve paralysis. J Bone Joint Surg 45A:1382, 1963.)

not pull the elbow proximally. A collar and cuff can easily be made out of 6-inch stockinet. Be sure to pad the neck area.

Definitive Treatment

Specific management depends on the fracture type, presence of associated injuries, and patient factors. Operative stabilization is generally favored in patients with multiple trauma, segmental fractures, and grossly unstable transverse fractures. In all other situations, many surgeons prefer to pursue closed management unless a delayed union or nonunion becomes obvious. Parameters for acceptable alignment are 20 degrees of anterior angulation, 30 degrees of varus and valgus angulation, and 3 cm of shortening.

Nerve Injury

Radial nerve dysfunction is sometimes noted in the ER when the patient with a humeral shaft fracture is first examined. In this situation, observation of the nerve injury is acceptable. It is critical to document nerve function before and after the patient is treated. This is because if the nerve palsy develops after a reduction maneuver, immediate operative exploration may be warranted.

Open fractures with nerve injury also usually require nerve exploration in addition to operative care of the fracture. Nerve palsies that are present from the outset can be observed for 3 to 4 months before exploration and neurolysis are considered. Usually electromyographic and nerve conduction velocity changes suggestive of recovery can be documented at 6 weeks, and if such recovery occurs, operative exploration is usually deferred in favor of continued observation.

SUPRACONDYLAR AND CONDYLAR HUMERAL FRACTURES

Clinical Assessment

Fractures in the distal metaphyseal region of the adult humerus commonly result from axial load with the elbow extended. The elbow is swollen, tender, and unstable. Physical exam will help in localizing the fracture, but identification of the exact type of humeral fracture can be very difficult without an x-ray. These patients will be labeled by the ER as having an "elbow fracture." Carefully assess neurovascular status. Radiographic evaluation will require the usual AP and lateral films, although because of instability of the elbow, an assistant may be required to hold the extremity while the x-ray technician takes the picture. Comparison views of the normal elbow and distal humerus may be helpful, although this is much more commonly required in pediatric elbow injuries.

Treatment Considerations

True isolated supracondylar fractures in adults are rare. More commonly, the fracture extends into the joint, creating the "T"-intercondylar-type fracture. Riseborough and Radin have classified the adult intercondylar fracture as follows (Fig. 4–3):

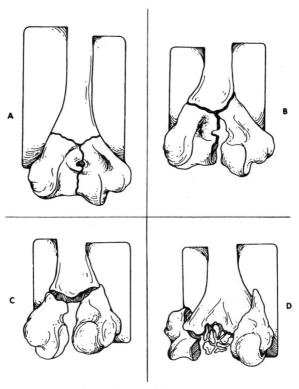

Figure 4–3. Adult distal humeral fractures. *(A)* Type I: nondisplaced T condylar; *(B)* Type II: displaced but not rotated; *(C)* Type III: displaced and rotated; *(D)* Type IV: displaced, rotated, and comminuted. (From Bryan, RS: Fractures about the elbow in adults. Instructional Course Lectures 30:200-223, 1981, by permission of Mayo Foundation.)

- Type I—undisplaced
- Type II—displaced without rotation of the fragments
- Type III—displaced and rotated
- Type IV—severely comminuted

If any displacement is present, surgery is usually necessary to anatomically realign the joint surface. An olecranon osteotomy to achieve exposure, and use of medial and lateral plates are often required to rigidly fix these unstable, articular fractures. Severely comminuted fractures can be a problem. In elderly patients, other treatment options include traction management or elbow arthroplasty.

Immediate care consists of a single, careful attempt at closed reduction and a long-arm splint (of course, assuming that neurovascular and soft-tissue compromise do not mandate emergency surgery). In most cases when the patient presents with significant malalignment, surgery is necessary to ensure an anatomic joint line and a reduction stable enough to allow early motion (within a few weeks).

Isolated Condylar Fractures

Isolated condylar fractures can also occur. Lateral condylar fractures are more common than medial, and both types are classified according to Milch:

- Type I—fracture through trochlea or capitellum with intact lateral trochlear ridge
- Type II—fracture involving a larger part of the distal humerus and extending through the lateral trochlear ridge

Condylar fractures are similar to the intercondylar-type supracondylar fractures in that they require anatomic reduction of the joint surface. If any displacement or articular step-off greater than 2 millimeters is present, open reduction and internal fixation will be necessary.

CAPITELLAR AND TROCHLEAR FRACTURES OF THE DISTAL HUMERUS

Clinical Assessment

The general presentation and exam features of patients with capitellar and trochlear fractures will be similar to those described in the previous section on distal humeral fractures. Because capitellar and trochlear fractures represent articular surface injuries, anatomic reduction is required. If initial displacement is present, rarely can these fragments be satisfactorily realigned by closed reduction. Limited soft tissue attaches to these fracture pieces, and consequently closed manipulation affords poor control.

Treatment Considerations

Fractures of the capitellum are more common than isolated trochlear fractures in adults. Capitellar fractures are classified into two types, depending on how much subchondral bone is present on the fracture fragment.

- Type I (Hahn-Steinthal) represents the capitellar articular surface and a large (usually hemispherical) segment of underlying cancellous bone. The fracture piece is often displaced anteriorly and malrotated by at least 90 degrees, wedged on top of the radial head. Open reduction is often necessary, followed by internal fixation with several screws (Fig. 4–4).
- Type II (Kocher-Lorenz) consists of just an articular shell with minimal subchondral bone; excision may be required for definitive treatment (see Fig. 4–4).

Immediate care in the ER consists of a single attempt at closed manipulation (but only if manipulation is judged to be worthwhile), followed by application of a long-arm splint and early office follow-up to plan definitive care.

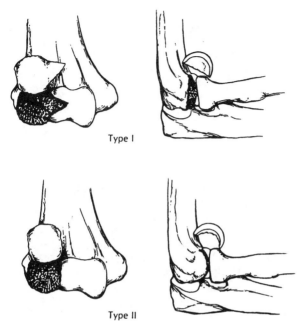

Type I

Type II

Figure 4–4. Capitellar fractures. The type I (Hahn-Steinthal) produces a capitellar fragment that contains some cancellous bone. The type II (Kocher-Lorenz) variant has almost no subchondral bone attached to the capitellar fragment, making this piece of "eggshell" cartilage very difficult to internally fixate. (From Rockwood, CA, Jr., Green, DP, and Bucholz, RW [eds]: Fractures in Adults. JB Lippincott, Philadelphia, 1991, p 769, with permission.)

OLECRANON AND CORONOID FRACTURES

Clinical Assessment

Olecranon fractures are very common, usually resulting from a fall on an extended forearm or a direct blow. Physical exam demonstrates tenderness and swelling over the proximal ulna. Because the bone is subcutaneous, a defect or instability can often be appreciated. Active extension of the elbow may dramatize loss of extensor mechanism continuity, but this demonstration is not often required to make the diagnosis and may actually cause further displacement of the fracture. Simple AP and lateral views of the elbow are typically sufficient to delineate the injury.

Coronoid process fractures are rare but merit some mention because, if present with other elbow injuries, they can contribute to severe elbow instability.

Treatment Considerations

Olecranon fractures can be classified into two basic groups: undisplaced and displaced. *Undisplaced olecranon fractures* may be treated with cast immobilization. Start with a long-arm posterior mold in the ER. Keep the elbow flexed only to about 70 degrees to relax the triceps' pull on the fracture fragment and obtain another x-ray once the splint is in place to confirm that no further displacement has occurred.

Displaced olecranon fractures typically require operation for two reasons: (1) the olecranon represents an articular surface that must be anatomically aligned, and (2) significant separation will result in some loss of active elbow extension. These fractures are typically fixed operatively within the first 5 to 7 days of injury.

Tension band wiring is a popular technique of internal fixation, but plates and screws may additionally be required depending on the obliquity of the fracture, degree of comminution, and distal extent of the fracture line. A fracture extending distal to the coronoid process usually requires a plate and starts to behave more like an ulnar shaft fracture.

When an elbow dislocation, radial head fracture, or olecranon fracture is present, take a look at the *coronoid process*. Although no acute care (other than splinting) is required, coronoid process involvement may be an ominous sign when the other periarticular or ligamentous injuries are present. Regan and Morrey have classified coronoid fractures into three types:

- Type I—tip avulsion

- Type II—less than 50 percent fractured
- Type III—more than 50 percent fractured

Type III fractures may require internal fixation, especially in the setting of additional elbow injury and gross instability.

RADIAL HEAD AND NECK FRACTURES

Clinical Assessment

Radial head and radial neck fractures are both common injuries in adults. Although the elbow shows apparently diffuse tenderness and swelling, direct, gentle thumb pressure over the radial head at the posterolateral elbow will elicit acute discomfort, especially with gentle passive pronation and supination. Occasionally, crepitance can be palpated with this maneuver, confirming the location of injury.

In addition to the standard AP and lateral views of the elbow, radiographic evaluation can be facilitated with a "radial head view," which is an oblique x-ray with the elbow at 90 degrees of flexion. This provides a nice profile of the radial head and neck. Nondisplaced radial head and neck fractures can sometimes be very difficult to diagnose; all that will be noted is diffuse elbow pain and a "fat pad sign" on the x-ray. In these cases, look very carefully for a crack in the radial head or a slightly impacted radial neck fracture; the radial head view can be invaluable.

Treatment Considerations

Radial head fractures have been classified by Mason into four types:

- Type I—nondisplaced
- Type II—single large displaced fragment
- Type III—comminuted
- Type IV—fracture with elbow dislocation

Definitive treatment for a type I fracture is early motion, and typically a simple sling is required for the first week. No plaster splint is necessary unless severe discomfort is encountered. The most common complication of a type I fracture is stiffness; usually, the sooner the patient moves the elbow and uses it functionally, the better.

A type II radial head fracture may require surgery. Although some debate continues about surgical indications, common guidelines include a fracture fragment representing 33 percent or more of the head, with 3 mm or more of displacement, and 30 degrees or more of angulation. Finding such a fracture without too much comminution to preclude stable fixation is rare.

Comminuted radial head fractures (type III) have been a topic of controversy. Many surgeons recommend excision, and the timing of excision (within 24 hours or beyond 2 weeks, or somewhere in between) has also been a topic of controversy. Be sure to communicate with your attending physician if the head is totally comminuted in the event that he or she prefers immediate excision (within 24 hours). Comminuted radial head fractures associated with medial elbow ligamentous disruption or other periarticular fractures (e.g., olecranon, coronoid process) may be part of an injury pattern that produces severe elbow instability.

In addition to addressing these other injuries, a Silastic radial head prosthesis may be an option for management of the radial head fracture (versus just excision). Use of a Silastic radial head or any type of radial head prosthesis is a topic of much debate and probably depends on the individual preferences of the surgeon and the specific situation.

Radial neck fractures are typically mildly or moderately impacted and, similar to type I radial head injuries, can be treated with a sling and an emphasis on early motion. If the neck fracture is angulated more than 30 degrees (and consequently produces noncongruous movement with forearm rotation), open reduction and/or internal fixation may be indicated. Remember that some "elbow sprains" are really minimally impacted radial neck fractures. Study the x-ray and follow the gentle subcapital cortical curvature of the radial head to confirm that there is no sudden break or step-off characteristic of a fracture.

RADIAL AND ULNAR SHAFT FRACTURES

Clinical Assessment

Patients with radial and ulnar shaft fractures present with obvious forearm deformity and instability. Nerve injuries can result from direct trauma to the nerve by bone fragments or by traction type trauma from the initial deformity. Remember that the original deformity may have been much worse than what the patient demonstrates in the ER, because the ER staff or paramedics have usually partially splinted or straightened the forearm.

When examining the patient, palpate the radial head or the distal ulnar regions to assess for tenderness. Sometimes, a radial head dislocation or distal ulnar dislocation associated with a forearm shaft fracture will have been fortuitously reduced by the time you first meet the patient. You must suspect such an occurrence if the x-rays show an isolated radial or ulnar shaft fracture, which is quite uncommon.

The patient with elbow or wrist tenderness with an ulnar or radial shaft fracture most likely has the Monteggia or Galeazzi injury pattern.

Radiographic Evaluation

Radiographic examination of radial and distal ulnar fractures requires *full-length AP and lateral views* of the forearm. These must include the elbow and wrist joints, especially if only one long bone is broken in the shaft.

The radius and ulna are mechanically interconnected by the interosseous membrane, and it is difficult to break only one bone without breaking or dislocating the other. Consequently, a radial head dislocation associated with an ulnar shaft fracture (Monteggia lesion) or a distal ulnar dislocation associated with a radial shaft fracture (Galeazzi fracture) can be missed unless the wrist and elbow are included in radiographic assessment. <AU5>The initial films obtained in the ER commonly *will not* include the appropriate adjacent joints. Be sure that the necessary films are obtained.

Fracture Classification

The Bado classification is popular for Monteggia lesions.

- Type I—anterior radial head dislocation
- Type II—posterior dislocation
- Type III—lateral dislocation of the radial head
- Type IV—anterior dislocation with both radial and ulnar shafts broken

The Galeazzi fracture is not subclassified, although the name *Piedmont* is also commonly used to describe this injury pattern.

Initial Treatment

Immediate treatment for either shaft fractures or the Monteggia or Galeazzi lesion consists of gently straightening the forearm and immobilizing it in a long-arm posterior mold. If the distal radial-ulnar joint or radial head is dislocated, this can usually be reduced simply with direct thumb pressure. Positioning the forearm at 90 degrees of flexion and in supination may help to hold either the distal ulnar or proximal radial dislocation. Be aware that *the definitive treatment in adults almost always requires operative internal fixation* and that reduction in the ER setting is primarily for comfort and reduction of soft-tissue tension (which unloads pressure on neurovascular structures and also reduces swelling).

Surgery is usually undertaken within a few days of the injury if soft-tissue compromise or multiple-trauma issues do not mandate immediate operation.

Definitive Treatment

If any displacement or angulation is present when shafts of both the radius and ulna are broken in adults, the bones must be internally fixed, usually with AO plates and screws. Note that in children, both bone fractures (including Monteggia and Galeazzi lesions) usually do *not* require surgery. What then is the age when treatment changes from nonoperative to operative? Although this is controversial, many authors believe that for girls older than 12 years and boys older than 14 years, forearm shaft fractures assume a more adult character and do better with surgery.

In the case of a Monteggia or Galeazzi lesion, the long-bone shaft involved (ulna or radius, respectively) must be internally fixed. Often, the associated dislocation can be simply closed reduced and held stable if the long-bone fracture is operatively fixed and the extremity splinted in a position of stability (elbow flexion for the most common Monteggia, forearm supination for Galeazzi).

Isolated Ulnar Fracture

An isolated ulnar shaft fracture can occur from a direct blow to the forearm. This is referred to as a "nightstick" fracture. Confirm that the radial shaft and the elbow and wrist are normal on physical and radiographic exam before accepting the nightstick diagnosis. This fracture can be definitively treated with a long-arm cast as long as there is no more than 10 degrees of angulation and no more than 50 percent displacement; otherwise, plate fixation is better.

Some authors have shown that for nondisplaced isolated ulnar shaft fractures, union can be achieved with a minimum of immobilization (removable brace, etc.), but this depends upon the personal preferences of the attending orthopaedic surgeon.

DISTAL RADIAL FRACTURES

Clinical Assessment

Distal radial fractures are among the most common fractures in adults, occurring in all age ranges. Falling on an outstretched arm is a typical mechanism. A neurovascular exam with respect to the median nerve is particularly important before any attempt at reduction. As usual, examine the wrist and elbow in addition to the forearm. For example, some radial fractures can occur in combination with scaphoid fractures or carpal ligamentous disruptions. A "dinner fork" appearance of the distal forearm is the classic deformity, which occurs as a result of dorsal displacement of the distal fragment.

The distal ulna is invariably injured as well and may present either as some type of fracture (ulnar styloid or ulnar neck) or as a ligamentous disruption (triangular fibrocartilage complex).

Fracture Eponyms

Colles's fracture is often applied to any type of distal radial fracture. To be technically correct, however, the name "Colles" specifically refers to a simple, metaphyseal distal radial fracture, with volar angulation and dorsal displacement of the distal fragment (Fig. 4–5).

Smith's fracture is a metaphyseal distal radial fracture with dorsal angulation and volar displacement (usually caused by a dorsal blow to a flexed wrist, the opposite mechanism of a Colles).

Barton's fracture refers to an intra-articular fracture, best demonstrated on a lateral x-ray, in which the volar margin of the distal radius is broken, allowing the carpus to sublux volarly.

Dorsal Barton's fracture occurs when the dorsal (or posterior) rim of the radius is broken, allowing the carpus to sublux dorsally.

Chauffeur's fracture refers to an intra-articular fracture in which the radial styloid has broken off in one large chunk; scapholunate dissociation is a frequent associated injury.

Radiographic Evaluation

Radiographic evaluation of distal radial fractures should consist of AP and lateral views; occasionally oblique views and comparison views of the uninjured side are helpful. The eponyms noted previously have strong historical roots but may not be helpful in describing a fracture to someone else, because the eponyms are used rather loosely and have different meanings to different people. There are also a multitude of classification systems (e.g., Frykman, Gartland and Werley, Melone, and May). Although it is useful to learn and under-

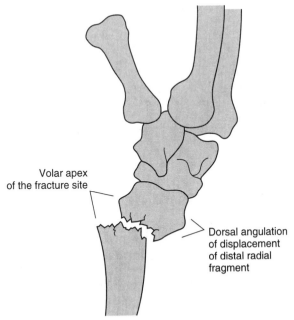

Volar apex
of the fracture site

Dorsal angulation
of displacement
of distal radial
fragment

Figure 4–5. A typical Colles-type distal radius fracture. Note the typical volar angulation and dorsal displacement of the fracture segment. (From McKinnis, LN: Fundamentals of Orthopedic Radiology. FA Davis, Philadelphia, 1997, p 413, with permission.)

stand these classification systems, probably the best way to describe a distal radial fracture over the phone or in a conference is to first describe objective fracture geometry (save discussion about the best eponym or classification for later), as in the following guidelines:

1. Mention whether the fracture is intra-articular or limited to the metaphysis; if intra-articular, mention whether the radiocarpal or ulnocarpal joints (or both) are involved.
2. Mention the quality of the bone and degree of comminution present.
3. Describe the position of the distal fragment relative to the radial shaft (angulation and displacement).

4. For both the prereduction and postreduction x-rays, note three features of alignment that determine acceptability: radial length, articular inclination (measured on an AP view), and palmar tilt (as seen on a lateral view). Ideally, one would like less than 5 mm of shortening and a minimal loss of articular inclination (normal = 22 degrees) and palmar tilt (normal = 11 degrees). A fourth critical factor that affects long-term outcome is articular congruity of the distal radius; ideally, one should strive for less than a 2-mm "step-off" or depression in the articular surface.

Treatment Considerations

Most distal radial fractures ultimately require only cast immobilization. Consequently, this fracture may represent the greatest opportunity for an orthopaedic resident to effect the definitive treatment. A simple closed-reduction attempt should probably be performed at least once in the ER for any significantly malaligned distal radial injury. With a little practice, these reduction maneuvers can become quite routine. If your postreduction films do not look acceptable, do not despair. This usually means that the fracture requires more than a cast to achieve or maintain a satisfactory position.

Closed Reduction and Cast Application

Depending on individual preference of the surgeon, a closed reduction can be performed just with bare hands or by using "Chinese finger trap" traction. A single bending maneuver with your bare hands might be all that is necessary for a slightly angulated, metaphyseal fracture. However, for all other fractures, the traps allow one to overcome the forces of forearm muscles in spasm (in both surgeon and patient) and also tend to realign smaller, intra-articular fragments better. Furthermore, use of traps is like having an assistant present; the traps hold the patient's extremity (and effect a traction-related reduction) while you ready the cast materials and organize the ER area.

Some form of anesthesia is required for reduction of a distal radial fracture. A hematoma block using 1 percent lidocaine is reliable. See Appendix D for the technique of hematoma block administration.

Many distal radial fractures can be reduced by placing the wrist in a position of moderate ulnar deviation (20 degrees) and mild flexion (20 degrees).

Keep in mind that some fractures, either because of fracture pattern (Barton's) or bone quality (severe osteopenia), cannot be adequately stabilized in plaster and subsequently require re-reduction or operative care. Carefully instruct the patient to follow up in the office within a few days. Be sure to discuss the importance of wrist elevation and gentle finger motion to reduce swelling. If a circumferential plaster bandage is applied in the ER, it is a good idea to split the cast dorsally with a cast saw before the patient is sent home.

CARPAL BONE FRACTURES

Clinical Assessment

Carpal bone fractures include a large spectrum of injuries, but the most common entity is probably the scaphoid fracture. Physical exam of any wrist injury should include careful palpation for the area of maximum tenderness. Although the wrist may seem like a small area, tenderness is usually localized to one region or another. Presence of ulnar and dorsal pain versus radial and volar pain will indicate two completely different diagnoses. Try to name the bone or structure closest to the tender spot; hamate fractures will be most tender over the hamate. Because most of the carpal bones have surfaces on both the dorsal and volar sides of the wrist, palpate both sides carefully and correlate any abnormal findings with anatomic landmarks. Note that for some ulnar carpal injuries, the ulnar nerve and artery can be compromised. If signs of ulnar artery thrombosis or ulnar nerve compromise exist, for example, be careful to assess for the presence of a hamate fracture or pisiform injury.

Scaphoid injuries usually demonstrate tenderness both in the "snuffbox" and volarly at the distal pole of the bone. The snuffbox is that region located at the dorsal aspect of the base of the thumb, between the first and second extensor tendon compartments. Subtle swelling may accompany these findings, and comparison with the appearance and sensitivity of the uninjured wrist can be helpful.

Radiographic Evaluation

In addition to AP and lateral views, a slightly oblique PA view in full ulnar deviation can be invaluable in identifying a scaphoid fracture. This view presents the scaphoid in a full profile and may demonstrate a crack that is otherwise invisible on routine films (Fig. 4–6). Other helpful views include a clenched fist AP and a radial deviation view. Do not forget that a true lateral view can diagnose a variety of severe derangements (in particular, carpal dislocations) and comparison with a lateral view of the normal side can be very revealing. Fractures involving the hook of the hamate may be best seen with a "carpal tunnel view."

Treatment Considerations

Keep the following management considerations in mind for treatment of carpal bone fractures:

1. Be careful not to miss a scaphoid injury. Because of its peculiar blood supply, scaphoid fractures can be notoriously troublesome, sometimes requiring inordinately long periods of time to heal or even requiring internal fixation and bone grafting to demonstrate union.
2. An unstable, ununited scaphoid can produce severe carpal instability and quite reliably yield a painful arthritic wrist. Furthermore, because many scaphoid fractures are difficult to visualize without special views or special imaging, it pays to carefully examine the patients in the ER. Any patient with tenderness in the snuffbox region or other physical or radiographic clues suggesting a scaphoid injury should be properly immobilized until the injury can be further defined. This means placing patients suspected of scaphoid injury in at least a forearm-based thumb

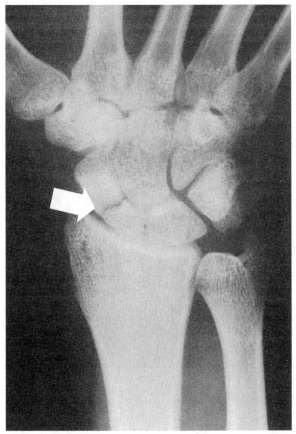

Figure 4–6. X-ray of a nondisplaced scaphoid fracture. (From Starkey, C, and Ryan, J: Evaluation of Orthopedic and Athletic Injuries. FA Davis, Philadelphia, 1996, p 428, with permission.)

spica-type splint or cast; some surgeons prefer a long-arm thumb spica for initial treatment of confirmed scaphoid fractures.
3. The prognosis of scaphoid injuries is related to the level and type of fracture. Proximal pole fractures have the highest nonunion rate (70 percent). Middle third fractures have a somewhat lower nonunion

rate (30 percent); distal third fractures usually heal consistently in about 6 weeks.

4. The presence of any displacement greater than 1 mm mandates a reduction, which typically requires surgery. A wide degree of displacement may dictate emergency surgery, because wide separation of the two fragments implies that the proximal fragment's blood supply is jeopardized.

5. A common avulsion fracture involves the triquetrum in which a flake of bone can be seen dorsal to the wrist on a lateral radiograph. Patients will be tender over the dorsal and ulnar wrist. This injury behaves like a sprain and usually can be treated with a splint or cast for 3 to 6 weeks.

METACARPAL FRACTURES

Clinical Assessment

The *most common location for a metacarpal fracture is the fifth metacarpal neck.* Called a "boxer's fracture," this injury occurs from striking a fixed object (such as a wall or another person's jaw) with a closed fist. Examine the hand closely for tenderness and instability, because multiple metacarpal fractures may be present. The base of the metacarpal (at the carpometacarpal articulation) is another area that sometimes fractures when a sudden axial load is applied.

Fractures of the metacarpal head and shaft usually occur from a direct blow (Fig. 4–7).

Additional points of the physical exam include checking for angulation and malrotation of the affected digits. This can be more subtle than it sounds, because with the digits extended, rotational and longitudinal malalignments may not be obvious. Ask the patient to gently allow the fingers to flex and compare both hands. In flexion, malrotation deformities become more noticeable; in the normal situation, all of the digits tend to line up evenly next to each other and all of the nailbeds point in the same general direction. In some people, the small finger normally curls under the ring finger; so compare the injured hand with the normal one. Any angulation or malrotation usually becomes obvious

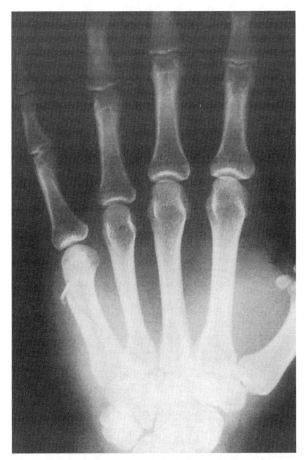

Figure 4–7. A fifth metacarpal shaft fracture. (From Starkey, C, and Ryan, J: Evaluation of Orthopedic and Athletic Injuries. FA Davis, Philadelphia, 1996, p 429, with permission.)

upon careful study of the injured hand with the digits flexed.

Radiographic examination consists of AP and lateral views. Occasionally, a 30-degree AP oblique film delineates more detail for the metacarpal head or metacarpal base.

Metacarpal Fractures with Bite Wounds

Soft-tissue considerations for metacarpal neck fractures deserve special mention. In the bar fight scenario (which is fertile ground for producing boxer's fractures), oftentimes the patient strikes another person in the jaw, not only fracturing the metacarpal neck, but also cutting the dorsal skin on his opponent's tooth. This "fight bite" usually represents an open laceration that extends down to bone. The hand is clenched when the injury occurs, and the metacarpophalangeal (MCP) joint of the affected finger is contaminated by a human bite. Unrecognized, *this can lead to a disastrous infection*, because human saliva is loaded with pathogens, and the MCP joint is a relatively closed space.

The bite wound itself appears innocuous at first and may be relatively small. When the MCP joints are held in extension (as they are when you are examining the hand), the laceration will not even look as if it is near the joint. Do not be fooled. Gently flex the MCP joint and watch how the skin moves. Checking a lateral x-ray may also be helpful; if you study the film carefully, sometimes a tooth-mark indentation can be seen directly in the metacarpal head.

Wound treatment consists of tetanus prophylaxis, appropriate antibiotic coverage (usually ampicillin/sulbactam [Unasyn], which covers gram-positive and gram-negative organisms, including a bug called *Eikenella corrodens*), and *open operative irrigation and débridement of the wound*. Before dismissing a metacarpal fracture (especially in intoxicated individuals), be sure that there are no soft-tissue complexities.

Treatment Considerations

Treatment of metacarpal fractures varies with the location of injury and degree of malalignment. Metacarpal neck fractures rarely require more than closed reduction and splinting for several weeks. Because of the mobility of the fifth metacarpal ray, dorsal angulation of up to 40 degrees can be accepted for a boxer's fracture. Closed manipulation in the ER followed by an ulnar gutter application (with plaster extending just past the MCP joint) is the usual course. Less angulation can be accepted for the other metacarpal necks; the rule is 30 degrees for the ring finger, 20 degrees for the long finger, and 10 degrees for the index finger, which is the least mobile ray, and therefore compensates the least well for a deformity.

Metacarpal Head and Shaft Fractures

Metacarpal head fractures can be treated with external splinting as long as there is no significant articular incongruity (less than 2 mm of step-off). Metacarpal shaft fractures also may not require operative care unless significant malrotation (more than 5 degrees), shortening (more than 5 mm), or angulation is present. Be aware that malrotation must be checked on physical exam; it will *not* be obvious on radiographic examination, especially for short oblique or spiral shaft fractures.

Metacarpal Base Fractures

Metacarpal base injuries can be serious injuries if the carpometacarpal (CMC) joint is involved. These intra-articular injuries usually involve more than just one ray and are often associated with significant CMC instability, requiring operative treatment. A particularly common metacarpal base fracture involves the thumb metacarpal, and is called *Bennett's fracture* (Fig. 4–8). This fracture pattern yields a small fragment of bone that stays in place, held by the volar oblique thumb ligament, while the rest of the thumb metacarpal shaft breaks free and displaces proximally. This fracture also routinely requires operative stabilization. These injuries are easy to underestimate because frequently only one radiographic view will clearly show the fracture, and, even so, a CT scan or tomogram is often necessary to clearly delineate the extent of the fracture. Studies reviewing the presentation of the CMC fracture dislocation note that it has a very high incidence of being missed on first examination, so be careful to suspect this injury pattern if metacarpal base tenderness and swelling correlates with an abnormal-appearing x-ray of this region.

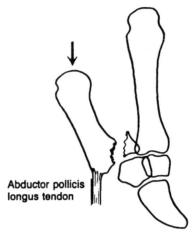

Abductor pollicis
longus tendon

Figure 4–8. A Bennett's fracture, or fracture dislocation of the thumb carpometacarpal joint. Note how the pull of the abductor pollicis longus tendon tends to displace the shaft proximally relative to the small articular fracture segment that remains at the joint line. (From Tsuge, K: Comprehensive Atlas of Hand Surgery. Nankodo Publishing, Tokyo, 1989, p 195, with permission.)

Multiple Metacarpal Fractures

This injury pattern represents a special circumstance. When a single metacarpal shaft is broken, the adjacent metacarpals exert a stabilizing effect through the deep transverse metacarpal ligament. However, if multiple adjacent metacarpals are fractured, significant instability of the hand can result. Multiple metacarpal shaft fractures routinely demand internal fixation to control rotation and angulation because the stabilizing effect of normal adjacent rays is lost.

PHALANGEAL FRACTURES

Clinical Assessment

Phalangeal fractures are usually caused by sports injuries or household trauma. It is helpful to inquire about the patient's occupation and hand dominance.

The physical exam should identify areas of tenderness and/or instability. Also, assess the skin for any lacerations (do not forget to check the web spaces). The general alignment of the digit should be checked because some fractures look perfectly reduced on x-ray but are actually significantly malrotated. In particular, rotational alignment of the fingers should be examined with the fingers flexed, because this accentuates any tendency for a malrotated finger to "crossover" an adjacent digit. Compare the injured hand with the noninjured hand, because many people normally demonstrate some overlap of the ring finger on the small finger. Simply ask the patient to rest both elbows on a table, keeping the forearms vertical and then allowing the fingers to gently curl into flexion. Even patients with multiple phalangeal or metacarpal fractures can tolerate this and it allows the examiner to view the fingertips on end; malrotation will be obvious either from gross crossover of fingers or just from the malrotated appearance of a fingernail.

Radiographic Evaluation

Assessment should include AP and lateral views. It is crucial to obtain true AP and lateral views, that is, views that are perpendicular to the bone and centered about the pathology. Management of hand fractures often depends on recognition of subtle fracture characteristics; features such as joint subluxation or articular surface fractures cannot be appreciated on partially oblique films. Do not accept inadequate x-rays.

Classification of phalangeal fractures is probably best accomplished by naming the involved bone (proximal, middle, or distal) and then describing the fracture geometry (e.g., transverse, oblique, angulated).

Distal Phalanx Fractures: Treatment Considerations

Most distal phalanx fractures are treated with external splinting, especially the common distal third or *tuft* fractures. An aluminum splint will do fine in the ER. Do not extend the splint past the proximal interphalangeal

(PIP) joint if there is no injury there; even an uninjured PIP joint will become stiff if immobilized. Distal phalanx *shaft* fractures occasionally require pinning if there is significant displacement or angulation. Fractures that occur from crushing mechanisms are quite tender, and splint immobilization provides protection and pain relief.

Periarticular fractures usually are the result of avulsion forces and infrequently require surgery. The most common such fracture is the "mallet finger," in which the extensor mechanism's terminal tendon is avulsed from the dorsal edge of the distal phalanx base. Treatment consists of extension splinting at the DIP joint.

Operative intervention for periarticular avulsion fractures is reserved for digits that manifest joint subluxation or an articular fragment that represents more than 40 percent of the joint surface (requires careful analysis of a true lateral view).

Fingertip Crush Injuries

Distal phalangeal crush injuries merit special mention because the fracture component is often accompanied by significant soft-tissue trauma. Nailbed lacerations and circular skin lacerations require careful repair. Be aware that a distal phalangeal fracture can produce a large nailbed laceration and in some sense qualify as an open fracture. Nailbed tissue may actually be stuck in the fracture site. The fracture must be reduced and the nailbed repaired (loupe magnification helps). The soft-tissue trauma makes the fracture even less stable and careful splint application is essential.

Be sure that the patient understands that severe crush injuries with bone and soft-tissue damage can take a long time to heal and may occasionally require later operative intervention to address nail deformity. Hypersensitivity and cold intolerance of the crushed fingertip may persist for up to 2 years after injury. Nailbed and fingertip lacerations are discussed in more detail in Chapter 8.

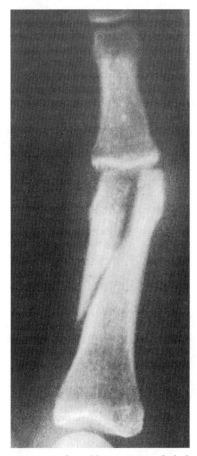

Figure 4–9. An x-ray of an oblique proximal phalangeal shaft fracture extending into the joint. Such fractures are predictably unstable, and the joint involvement mandates anatomic reduction. (From Starkey, C, and Ryan, J: Evaluation of Orthopedic and Athletic Injuries. FA Davis, Philadelphia, 1996, p 431, with permission.)

Proximal and Middle
Phalanx Fractures

Many fractures of the proximal and middle phalanges can also be satisfactorily treated with external immobilization. However, look carefully for any angulation or malrotation; these features are associated with unstable fractures that may do better with operative stabilization. The following are examples of unstable fractures:

- Long oblique shaft fractures (tend to rotate and shorten) (Fig. 4–9)
- Transverse midshaft fractures (tend to volarly angulate)
- Phalangeal neck fractures (phalangeal head portion displaces dorsally and rotates)

Any intra-articular fracture with more than 1 mm of step-off or diastasis usually requires operative correction. For angulated or malrotated digits, an attempt at closed reduction is certainly worthwhile; this involves manually correcting whatever clinical deformity is present. A digital block with local anesthetic may make the reduction process easier. Splint stabilization of the injured finger is frequently aided by "buddy" taping adjacent uninjured fingers to the injured digit.

Follow-up Instructions for
Hand Fractures

Emphasize to patients with hand injuries that *follow-up should be within a few days*. Phalangeal fractures heal quickly, and the injuries of those patients who return to the orthopaedist's office 2 weeks after injury have already almost healed. This makes management of unstable or malaligned fractures more difficult. Hand fracture patients also tend to acquire significant stiffness at adjacent joints and adjacent fingers, and *early* involvement of a hand therapist can be helpful. The therapist also can usually fabricate a custom-designed thermoplastic splint that is lighter and less cumbersome than a plaster or aluminum splint.

5
CHAPTER

Lower-Extremity Fractures

This chapter is a continuation of the previous chapter, now focusing on the major lower-extremity fractures. The main issues addressed here relate to the fundamentals of history, physical assessment, and initial management.

PROXIMAL FEMORAL (HIP) FRACTURES

Hip fractures represent one of the most common of all adult fractures, accounting for at least half of all hospital days related to fracture care in the United States. The two main varieties are *femoral neck* (intracapsular) and *intertrochanteric* fracture. In both cases, the patients are frequently elderly persons and have sustained injury from a fall at home or similar low-energy trauma. Factors that often contribute to falls in the elderly include physical hazards in the home environment, such as rugs, stairs, and electrical cords; the use of sedating medication; and the presence of poor balance or impaired vision.

Clinical Assessment

History

Determine the following information in taking the patient's history.

1. Obtain a history of how the injury occurred and, in particular, whether the fall was witnessed by anyone other than the patient. Establish whether the patient fell because of a loss of consciousness, because this would merit a cardiac and neurologic work-up in addition to caring for the orthopaedic injury.
2. Include the usual review of medication use and major medical problems. Be sure to ascertain whether the patient was ambulatory before the fall and to what degree.
3. Inquire whether the patient lives alone, with a spouse, or in a supervised care environment.
4. Determine the patient's mental status. This is a critically important element that can characterize the recovery course. You may need to rely on the patient's family or friends to get an accurate view of the preinjury functional status. A patient who is a debilitated, disoriented, nursing home resident presenting with a fractured hip has a very different prognosis from that of the patient with a hip fracture who is an independent ambulator, lives with his or her spouse, and leads an active lifestyle.

Physical Exam

The physical exam typically reveals that the injured leg is externally rotated and shortened compared with the normal side. These findings are usually obvious. Any motion of the injured extremity will produce severe pain centered about the affected groin. Examine the pelvic bony prominences for tenderness because occasionally pubic ramus fractures may also be present or confused with hip injury.

Document the presence of lower-extremity pulses (easily checked at the ankle) and neurologic function of the limb. Do not forget to assess the limb for any other areas of tenderness or deformity, because hip fractures can also present in combination with other fractures, such as those of the femur, tibia, or ankle.

Radiographic Assessment

The best films to obtain are an AP view of the pelvis in addition to AP and "shoot-through" lateral views of the affected hip.

1. The AP view of the pelvis will prevent you from missing an obvious contralateral hip injury and also provide a normal side by which to assess the injured hip.
2. The AP and lateral films of the affected side provide better exposure of the whole proximal femur and bone detail.
3. A shoot-through lateral film is better than a "frog" lateral film. A frog lateral film involves twisting the leg into further external rotation to obtain the film, whereas a shoot-through lateral film leaves the injured limb alone and relies on moving the x-ray beam to get a true lateral view of the proximal femur. Be aware that you may need to help the radiology technician hold the normal thigh up to obtain the shoot-through film. The shoot-through lateral view is the only film that accurately shows whether posterior angulation or comminution is present—important details in some situations.

The type of hip fracture can be immediately characterized by the radiographic appearance. Intracapsular fractures are those that involve the femoral neck, whether the break is immediately beneath the femoral head (subcapital) or just proximal to the intertrochanteric region (basilar neck). Intertrochanteric type injuries will show a fracture line that extends from the greater trochanter to the lesser trochanter.

Fracture Classification

In addition to describing what portion of the femoral neck is broken (subcapital versus basilar), femoral neck fractures are most commonly graded according to *Garden's fracture classification*, which characterizes the degree of displacement as seen on an AP hip film.

- Type I—incomplete crack through the femoral neck
- Type II—complete nondisplaced fracture
- Type III—displaced up to 50 percent of the neck diameter
- Type IV—displaced more than 50 percent of the neck diameter

Type I and II fractures are associated with a better rate of healing and reduced risk of developing osteonecrosis of the femoral head.

A variety of systems are used to classify intertrochanteric fractures, but almost all depend on whether the lesser and greater trochanter are separate pieces. A simple two-part fracture produces a distal shaft segment and a proximal head and neck piece. Three-part fractures show that the lesser trochanter has broken off as a separate segment, and four-part intertrochanteric fractures involve a shaft segment, head and neck segment, and the greater and lesser trochanters as separate additional pieces.

Hospital Admission

Patients with hip fracture must be admitted because they cannot walk and usually require surgery within 24 hours. Identify who will be the internist and contact that physician as soon as you have finished evaluating the patient. The internist typically must "clear" the patient as being medically stable for surgery, and the sooner you get the medical assessment process started, the more likely it is that surgery will not be delayed. Sometimes the patient is sick enough that a variety of tests may be necessary before surgery can be safely undertaken. However, most patients' condition can be optimized within 24 to 48 hours, and any further delay in stabilizing the hip often works against the patient's overall well-being.

Write an order for the patient to be placed in 5 to 10 lbs of "Buck's" traction when he or she arrives on the orthopaedic floor from the emergency room (ER). This type of traction is simply a foam boot that wraps around the ankle of the injured limb and attaches by a rope to a weight hanger at the foot of the bed. Five pounds of traction tends to gently pull the injured leg just enough that the patient cannot move it easily. This provides reasonable pain relief while the patient awaits surgery.

Surgical Treatment

Rarely does a hip fracture not mandate surgical management. Occasionally in a very debilitated patient who was previously bedridden and demented, a decision may be made in cooperation with the patient's family or guardian to leave the fracture alone. However, even in the nonambulatory patient, surgical fixation or arthroplasty (depending on fracture type) is often the best choice to provide pain relief and allow limb mobility for hygiene maintenance. Furthermore, operative management typically allows mobilization of the patient the day after surgery, and early mobilization is a profoundly positive influence on the patient's overall medical status. Remaining at bedrest for an extended period with a painful hip, on the other hand, greatly increases the risks of pulmonary compromise, skin breakdown, and other complications that often doom the patient to great morbidity and even death.

Internal Fixation

Nondisplaced femoral neck fractures often can be internally fixed with long, metal cannulated screws. Displacement of the femoral neck (Garden III or IV fractures) is associated with a much higher incidence of femoral head osteonecrosis, and consequently these fractures are usually better managed with prosthetic replacement (hemiarthroplasty). Be aware that the patient with a nondisplaced femoral neck fracture should be kept as immobile as possible until surgical fixation is achieved so that the fracture does not become displaced and thereby require a more extensive operation with a potentially worse prognosis. In younger patients, a closed reduction is often recommended in an attempt to save the patient's femoral head. The exact age at which internal fixation is deferred in favor of prosthetic replacement is somewhat controversial. Most surgeons will choose prosthetic replacement if the patient is between 65 and 75 years old, especially if the patient is less active or has other chronic illnesses. In very young patients, it is optimal to save the femoral head if at all possible and consequently the displaced femoral neck fracture in a younger adult represents a surgical emergency, because the length of time that the fracture is displaced increases the likelihood of osteonecrosis. These patients are treated urgently with an immediate attempt at closed reduction and surgical fixation in the operating room.

Intertrochanteric fractures are usually managed with internal fixation because the blood supply in this region is excellent and healing is more predictable. The most common form of fixation is a large threaded lag screw, which purchases the femoral head and mates distally into a side plate that is screwed onto the femoral shaft. This screw and side-plate device allows the fracture to settle in the postoperative period without forcing the lag screw to necessarily cut out of the bone, because the lag screw can slide through the side plate as the fracture construct shortens.

FEMORAL FRACTURES

In young patients with good bone stock, fractures of the femur often occur from high-energy trauma. Similar to patients with unstable pelvic fractures, patients with femoral fractures must be thoroughly assessed for other injuries and monitored for the physiological side effects of large-bone trauma.

Clinical Assessment

History

The history should document how the injury occurred and characterize whether it was a high-energy or low-energy trauma.

Physical Exam

The physical exam should include a screening assessment for other injuries. Do not assume that the limb with the broken femur cannot have another fracture present elsewhere (e.g., hip, knee, ankle, foot). Femoral shaft fractures can account for several units of blood loss into the thigh musculature very quickly, and this may account for the massive swelling seen around the fracture site. The limb is often grossly unstable, and any motion at the fracture site will produce terrific pain.

Traction

After documenting the neurovascular status of the limb, the extremity should be immobilized. This may be best accomplished with some form of traction, because application of a splint is difficult and ineffective for all but the most distal of femur fractures. If definitive surgical stabilization will be performed within 24 hours, sometimes Buck's traction (5 or 10 lb) is simplest and noninvasive. However, for any delay longer than 1 day, skeletal traction is best. Furthermore, in some situations, skeletal traction may be the definitive method of managing the fracture. In adults, the traction pin is usually placed in the proximal tibia. Discuss the initial management with your attending physician first before placing a traction pin, because sometimes the pin's presence may influence (perhaps negatively) subsequent options in treating the fracture.

Radiographic Assessment

A good AP and lateral x-ray of the fracture will allow proper assessment of the injury geometry. Be certain to obtain films that show the *entire* femur, from hip to knee. This means the AP and lateral films should show the proximal tibia in femoral fractures that are distal. This can be critically important in distal femoral fractures because sometimes the fracture will spiral all the way down to the distal femur and actually enter the joint. This articular extension will specifically influence the treatment options, because the joint surface alignment must be perfect to reduce the future likelihood of posttraumatic arthritis at the knee.

Be particularly careful to screen the hip joint for fracture. About 5 percent of femoral shaft fractures are associated with an ipsilateral femoral neck fracture, and both fractures usually require specific operative fixation.

As already noted, patients with fractures of the femur have grossly unstable extremities and are in a lot of pain with any movement. Therefore, it may be most expeditious (and humane) if you assist the radiology technician in positioning the limb while obtaining the x-rays.

Treatment

Treatment depends mostly on the location of the fracture and the general health and activity level of the patient. The three main areas of fracture are the subtrochanteric area, the shaft, and the supracondylar zone.

Subtrochanteric Fractures

Subtrochanteric fractures are treated much the same way as hip fractures. Traction is generally a very poor choice with respect to comfort, convenience, and the inevitable complications of prolonged immobility. Operative stabilization, therefore, is pursued in almost all situations. The type of fixation is different than in hip fractures, however, because with a more distal fracture location, the biomechanics of stabilization are different. Probably the best mechanical choice for internal fixation is an intramedullary rod, although occasionally a long plate that fixes proximally into the femoral head and neck may be used.

Femoral Shaft Fractures

The overwhelming choice for treating closed femoral shaft fractures is an intramedullary rod. Other choices such as traction, plating, or external fixation are also considerations, with the last alternative being more reasonable if the fracture is a severe open injury. However, an intramedullary rod provides excellent stability and typically allows for immediate mobilization of the patient, a detail generally characterizing lessened morbidity in the postinjury period. Furthermore, there are some data to suggest that "rodding" the fracture within the first 24 hours postinjury greatly reduces the overall rate of pulmonary and other organ-system complications. The type of rod used and how it is fixed (or "locked") above and below the fracture site depends upon the specific geometry and location of the fracture.

Supracondylar Fractures

Fractures through the distal femur, or supracondylar area, also typically do best with aggressive internal fixation if any significant malalignment is present. Fixation devices here include large plate and lag screw combinations as well as intramedullary rods with multiple locking screws. The major focus in treating supracondylar fractures is achieving anatomic alignment at the knee joint.

Traction

Keep in mind that skeletal traction can be used as the definitive treatment for almost any fracture of the femur. Traction can be very labor intensive and requires prolonged inpatient hospitalization. However, in some situations where the patient's bone quality is terrible, the fracture geometry is extremely unstable, or the patient's medical status somehow prohibits surgery, traction may be an excellent option. Placement of the traction pin is critical because the pin itself represents relative contamination of the medullary canal and may be less desirable if surgery is anticipated to follow shortly. Furthermore, if skeletal traction is chosen as the main modality of treatment, the pin should be placed as precisely as possible to reduce the likelihood of early loosening, skin complications, or infection.

Setting up skeletal traction is actually not particularly difficult but can be confusing the first few times you try it. If your attending physician decides to use skeletal traction, either just for the first 24 hours of admission or as the definitive treatment, it can be very helpful to contact the orthopaedic ward technician or nurse manager. Most hospitals will have such a person available, and they can be invaluable in helping you set up a standard "balanced traction" array on an orthopaedic bed.

PATELLAR FRACTURES

The patella is the largest sesamoid bone in the body. Fracture can occur either from a direct blow or from a sudden extension force (pulling the patella apart).

Clinical Assessment

Patients will present with a tense, tender knee effusion, and often you can palpate a defect in the patella itself. The patient will be unable to perform a straight-leg raise, although this will also be true if the quadriceps or patellar tendon is ruptured.

Radiographic Assessment

X-rays will demonstrate whether a patellar fracture is present or why extensor mechanism continuity has been lost. Even if the patella is not broken, tendon rupture can often be distinguished by x-ray, because quadriceps rupture will cause the patella to ride "low" from its normal position (patella baja), and patellar tendon failure will give rise to the high-riding patellar position (patella alta).

Anteroposterior and lateral films of the knee usually will provide enough information to diagnose the injury pattern. Occasionally, if the patellar fracture is a nondisplaced vertical line, a "sunrise" view, which is taken with the knee flexed 90 degrees, will show the pathology best. Injuries that are simple two- or three-part fractures represent lower-energy damage than comminuted stellate fractures. In the high-energy situation, be sure to check the proximal tibia and femoral condyles for associated fracture.

Treatment Considerations

Because the patella constitutes part of the articular contact surface within the knee joint, any significant malalignment requires correction. Displacement of more than 3 mm or an articular step-off of more than 2 mm generally mandates surgical intervention. The ease with which surgical fixation is accomplished may be related to the fracture geometry. High-energy fracture patterns, such as stellate fractures, can be very difficult to reconstruct and may sometimes require partial or complete excision of the bony fragments. Two-part transverse fractures, on the other hand, can be routinely fixed by several standard methods, such as tension band wiring or screw fixation (Fig. 5–1). Surgical management also typically includes repair of the extensor retinaculum, which is the surrounding fascial structure that is almost always torn when the patella breaks. In some situations in which the patient is very

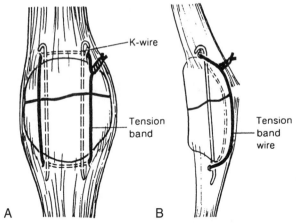

Figure 5–1. *(A)* Anteroposterior and *(B)* lateral diagrams of a typical transverse patellar fracture treated with tension-band wiring technique. (From Schatzker, J, and Tile, M [eds]: The Rationale of Operative Fracture Care. Springer-Verlag, Toronto, 1987, p 277, with permission.)

old, has poor bone quality, and presents with a comminuted fracture, complete excision of the patella with advancement of the quadriceps tendon may be the best solution for restoring knee extensor mechanism continuity.

Surgical management is usually scheduled within 1 week or less of the injury date. Until that time, a well-padded, bulky long-leg dressing with a knee immobilizer brace or splint will help reduce swelling and immobilize the knee for comfort and protection of the fracture position.

PROXIMAL TIBIAL FRACTURES

Proximal tibial fractures are common injuries that represent disruption of the tibia's support surface for the femoral condyles. They can occur from axial load of the knee joint or from a varus or valgus stress applied across the joint, or from a combination of angular load and axial compression. The lateral plateau is more commonly involved than the medial one, although both sides of the proximal tibia may be involved together. As the injury severity (energy transfer) increases, comminution and extension distally to involve the tibial metaphysis and shaft increase. The peak incidence for tibial plateau fractures in men is the fourth decade. Women are more likely to suffer a lower-energy injury in which poor bone quality plays a role in fracture occurrence. Injury mechanisms include falls, motor vehicle crashes, and sports injuries.

Clinical Assessment

Patients present with a tender effusion of the knee joint. Crepitance and instability of the proximal tibia is often evident on direct physical exam. Palpate the knee joint medially and laterally to check for tender or swollen areas around the knee collateral ligaments. These structures are commonly damaged with severe varus or valgus loading injuries. Be sure to document the neurovascular status of the limb and the tenseness of the soft tissues because compartment syndrome can occur from this fracture. If there is any doubt, measure compartment pressures (see Appendix B and Chapter 1). Injury to the popliteal artery is more common with a knee dislocation, but it can occur in some cases of severe plateau fractures.

Radiographic Assessment

Anteroposterior and lateral films of the knee are adequate for initial assessment of a proximal tibial fracture. Determine which plateau is involved (or both) and how much compression is present at the joint line. Treatment options depend upon the degree of articular step-off and joint-surface disruption. The lateral film will help visualize the posterior surface of the plateaus, which may be compressed to a variable degree depending upon the position of the knee when the injury occurred.

In many situations, additional imaging will be required to critically analyze the degree of joint-line disruption. Trispiral tomography used to be the standard for subsequent imaging, but these machines are less and less available. Usually, a computed tomography (CT) scan is performed, which will yield at least two planes of assessment and help resolve fracture lines to within 1 mm of displacement.

Treatment Considerations

After initial assessment in the ER, patients should be wrapped in a bulky padded long-leg bandage supported with a brace or plaster splint so that the knee cannot bend or shift in varus-valgus alignment. If gross deformity is present initially, the splint can be applied to achieve a "ballpark" correction of the deformity. Patients may then be referred for more sophisticated imaging if necessary (CT scan can be accomplished without removing the splint). In cases where energy transfer to the limb is low, patients may be sent home as long as they are carefully instructed in fracture and splint care, can independently maneuver without putting weight on the injured leg, and understand that they must return if severe pain persists. High-energy fractures (high comminution, involvement of the tibial metaphysis or both plateaus) are better managed with hospital admission and work-up. Severe plateau fractures can produce significant skin compromise and compartment syndrome, so do not hesitate to admit the patient if you are worried about the injury severity or the patient's reliability and self-care competence.

Definitive surgical management, when indicated, is often accomplished within 1 week of the injury date. Patients who meet the criteria for closed management (minimal step-off or malalignment) may be placed into a long-leg or cylinder cast, although usually the cast must be changed within the first few weeks as swelling decreases.

Nonsurgical Management

Nonsurgical care is adequate if the joint-line depression is 3 mm or less, if there is less than 5 mm of articular diastasis (widening), and if there is lateral tilt of 5 degrees or less. Deformity that exceeds these criteria is associated with a greater incidence of posttraumatic knee arthritis, and in the stable, ambulatory patient, surgical intervention is usually chosen to improve these odds. Most tibial plateau fracture classification systems describe the injury as involving the medial plateau, a central depressed segment, the lateral plateau, or a combination (Table 5–1).

Surgical Management

Surgical care focuses on restoration of the joint surface. In many situations, arthroscopic assessment of the knee joint can be performed while fracture segments are manipulated through another incision. The arthroscopy allows excellent visualization as the fragments are maneuvered into anatomic position. Often bone graft is then applied underneath the elevated segments to support their position. Internal fixation is then added, either with large screws to support elevated fracture pieces, or with large plates, which provide an even better buttress to hold sections of proximal tibia in place and squeeze the articular surface pieces together. The amount of internal fixation and type of plates or screws required depends on the comminution and geometry of the fracture.

Table 5–1. SCHATZKER CLASSIFICATION OF TIBIAL PLATEAU FRACTURES

Schatzker Type	Fracture Description
Type I	Wedge fracture of lateral plateau
Type II	Wedge fracture combined with depression of adjacent weight-bearing portion of lateral plateau
Type III	Central depression of lateral plateau without a lateral wedge component
Type IV	Fracture of the medial plateau
Type V	Bicondylar involvement: wedge fracture of medial and lateral plateaus
Type VI	Plateau fracture with separation of the tibial metaphysis from the diaphysis

Additional consideration must be given to collateral ligament disruptions that frequently accompany fractures about the knee. Medial collateral ligament damage is often present in concert with a lateral plateau fracture (valgus stress injury), and operative repair of the ligament, if indicated, may be accomplished at the same time as fracture fixation. Postoperatively, patients usually must protect the knee from weight bearing for 3 months or more, because undue compression before healing may crush the fracture segments again.

TIBIAL SHAFT FRACTURES

Tibial shaft fractures encompass a wide variety of patterns, depending upon the mechanism and severity of injury. They represent the most common of long-bone fractures in the United States.

Clinical Assessment

History

Establish whether the mechanism of injury was one of direct contact, twisting, bending, or axial load.

Physical Exam

Significant deformity is quite obvious because most of the bone anterior border is subcutaneous. Neurovascular assessment of the limb should focus on function of the peroneal (superficial and deep branches), anterior tibial, and posterior tibial nerves. Dorsalis pedis and posterior tibial arterial pulses must be checked carefully at the ankle. The status of the soft tissues is critically linked to management of the fracture. Note any lacerations, abrasions, compartment tension, or any other evidence of soft-tissue compromise.

Radiographic Assessment

The standard films are AP and lateral views of the entire tibia, including the knee and ankle joints. Additional imaging is usually not necessary. The fracture pattern should be described with respect to displacement, angulation, and comminution.

High-energy injuries (such as car bumper crushing accidents) show severe comminution, wide displacement of fracture pieces, and sometimes even segmental fractures patterns in fractures in which the tibial shaft is broken in two places. These can be highly treacherous injuries, producing compartment syndrome as well as being associated with prolonged healing times and residual deformity.

Lower-energy patterns include a single oblique or transverse fracture line with only mild or moderate displacement or angulation. Even in these injuries, however, the leg's anterior skin and soft-tissue envelope can be damaged or torn (producing an open fracture) because the anterior tibial margin is so subcutaneous.

Note where the fibula is broken. The fibula must be injured somewhere if the tibia is significantly fractured. If the fibula is broken at the same level as the tibia fracture, it makes the leg even more unstable. Occasionally, the fibula is broken obliquely at some distance from the tibial fracture level. A rotational force may break the tibia at one level, travel proximally as it crosses the interosseous membrane, and then exit the leg by breaking the fibula closer to the knee. Full-length films of the leg are necessary because the fibular injury can be easily missed with inadequate x-rays.

Treatment Considerations

Although tibial shaft fractures do not involve a joint surface, and therefore do not carry quite the same burden of anatomic alignment as an articular fracture, their treatment can be extremely difficult. Rotational deformity, shortening of the leg, and angular deformities can account for residual impairment in ambulation. Furthermore, definitive healing of the fracture is intimately linked with the status of the surrounding soft tissues, and disastrous problems such as infection or nonunion (or the catastrophic infected non-union) are unfortunately common as the severity of the soft-tissue and bony damage increases.

Casting

Most low-energy tibial shaft fractures can be definitively managed with a long-leg cast. Even so, in some situations, operative intervention may be chosen if only to allow the patient to weight-bear more quickly. Acceptable parameters for reduction include less than 1 cm of total shortening, less than 10 degrees of residual varus-valgus or flexion-extension angulation, and less than 20 degrees of residual external rotation and 10 degrees of residual internal rotation.

Surgery

Operative management for these fractures has included just about every possible method of fixing a bone. Plating was more popular many years ago, but because of the additional compromise caused by surgical stripping of the soft-tissue envelope, plating is probably the least favorite method of internal fixation today. Intramedullary rodding is perhaps the most common method of internally stabilizing an operative tibial shaft fracture today. External fixators offer another solution and are often the preferred modality in severe open fractures.

Special Problems and Complications

Tibial shaft fractures are perhaps the most common source of traumatic *compartment syndrome*. You must carefully assess the soft tissues when the patient presents, and for those fractures that represent high-energy trauma, admission to the hospital is warranted solely to monitor for potential compartment syndrome. If a long-leg cast is applied, splint it lengthwise or even bivalve it so that pressure build-up can be relieved and so that you can directly assess the leg by inspection and palpation without having to completely remove the cast. If you suspect that compartment syndrome is present, complete removal of the cast or splint (including the cast padding) must be performed, and compartment pressures should be measured. Segmental tibial fractures are notorious for producing compartment syndrome. Compartment syndrome is discussed in more detail in Chapter 1.

Application of a long-leg cast or splint is often necessary in the ER no matter what definitive treatment ultimately is indicated. Unless the fracture is an open one or the patient has multiple trauma, operative care is often not pursued immediately. Therefore, some sort of cast or splint is required even if the patient is destined for surgical care. Furthermore, most tibia fractures can be definitively managed with a cast anyway, so you will find yourself in a position to cast many of these injuries.

If it is clear that plaster immobilization is going to be temporary, use of a padded plaster splint (posterior mold) should suffice. Alternatively, it may be easier and much more secure to apply a regular long-leg cast and then just widely bivalve the cast or even remove the anterior half to ensure the swelling of the leg can be accommodated.

Placement of a long-leg cast can be difficult unless you have an assistant to help hold the leg. It may be helpful to first apply the short-leg component and let it dry for 5 minutes while you manually hold the reduction. Then the cast can be extended up above the knee without the fracture becoming completely unstable. The knee is best flexed about 30 degrees, and some plantar flexion of the ankle may relax the posterior calf muscles, allowing correction of the fracture's posterior angulation. Use your palms to mold the cast around the patella and supracondylar area of the distal femur, because a good fit here helps prevent the cast from sliding distally over time.

DISTAL TIBIAL PLAFOND FRACTURES

Injuries to the distal tibial plafond are called *pilon fractures,* so named as a description of the talus driving proximally into the distal tibial plafond like a hammer. The mechanism of injury is characteristically an axial load, often from a fall off a ladder. Associated injuries are therefore common because the energy involved is high. Other orthopaedic problems include calcaneus fracture, femoral or tibial shaft fractures, or vertical shear fractures of the pelvis.

Clinical Assessment

Pilon fractures demonstrate severe swelling and crepitance about the distal tibia, and based solely upon the physical exam, it may be hard initially to differentiate this injury from a more routine, lower-energy ankle fracture. Document the status of the neurovascular bundles to the ankle and the status of the surrounding skin.

Radiographic assessment begins with routine AP, lateral, and oblique films of the distal tibia. It is common that additional imaging is required to better assess the details of joint alignment. A CT scan is typically the favored modality. The critical features of reduction include articular step-off and overall parallelism between the distal tibial plafond and corresponding superior talar surface.

Treatment Considerations

Pilon fractures almost always require surgery unless there is near perfect alignment. An articular step-off of 2 mm or more is associated with development of posttraumatic ankle arthritis, so management relates to improvement of fracture alignment to at least this degree or better. Similar to tibial fractures, the soft-tissue status is the key determinant of when surgery is undertaken and how fracture fixation is approached. Pilon fractures are notorious for the swelling and skin blistering that they can produce, so if surgery is not undertaken within the first 12 hours postinjury, it is usually delayed for 7 to 10 days until swelling has improved.

The principles of operative care relate to four basic principles, as described by the Swiss fracture pioneers of the 1960s:

1. Internal fixation of the fibula, which restores the appropriate length parameter to the ankle joint
2. Reassembly of the tibial plafond articular fragments to restore a smooth, even joint surface
3. Insertion of bone graft proximal to the plafond to fill in the gap created by the crushing injury and to act as support to the restored articular surface

4. Consideration of the medial portion of the tibia for plating to provide a buttress that prevents the plafond from widening and impacting further

The key consideration in any surgical approach is the soft-tissue envelope. Many clinicians try to avoid exposing or extensively stripping the distal tibia because compromise of the soft tissues can lead to a disastrous cascade of tissue necrosis, fracture exposure, infection, and nonunion. Some more recently developed external fixators are designed to realign and stabilize the larger tibial fragments without mandating a major, open exposure. Some of the external fixators are strong enough to allow early weight bearing. The exact style of internal fixation for any given case will be dependent upon the soft-tissue status, fracture stability, and surgeon preference.

Initial ER care will typically not be dependent on the definitive treatment path. A long-leg plaster splint should be applied to control ankle motion and rotation. The skin should be prepped with iodine paint solution, because blistering inside the splint is not uncommon within the first few days after injury. Patients with anything more than a nondisplaced simple fracture should be admitted for ankle elevation, additional imaging (CT scan), and compartment syndrome monitoring.

FIBULAR FRACTURES

Clinical Assessment

Fibular shaft fractures can present as an isolated injury (from a direct blow) or present as part of a larger fracture pattern, such as an ankle injury or tibial shaft fracture. It is important to identify a reasonable explanation for how the fibula broke, because in some situations, the fibula may be the only obvious clue that a more serious injury is present. For example, with certain ankle fractures, the ligaments may be disrupted enough to produce severe instability medially, although the fibula is broken very proximally near the knee. Ankle films alone appear normal, but the high fibular fracture is a tip-off that an external rotation-type injury is present below. Therefore, be sure to examine the entire leg when the fibula is fractured, especially palpating the ankle. Any swelling or tenderness should be carefully assessed for its possible relationship to the fibula. A swollen ankle merits palpation of the fibula from ankle to knee, and any suspected findings on examination merit inclusion of full-length fibular films in addition to the routine ankle views.

Treatment Considerations

Fibular fractures not associated with ankle injury rarely require any specific treatment. Treatment of the tibial fracture will concomitantly allow the fibula to heal. An isolated fibular shaft fracture caused by a direct blow can often be treated just with an elastic bandage to reduce swelling. The management of fibular fractures in association with ankle injuries will be discussed later.

ANKLE FRACTURES

Ankle fractures are in the same company as hip and wrist injuries in that they are among the most common major fracture patterns that you will see in the ER. The mechanism of injury in most situations is either an external rotation or severe abduction force applied across the joint. Usually, the foot is planted firmly and the patient's leg (and body) twists or bends suddenly and the ankle (bone or ligament or both) fails.

Clinical Assessment

Patients present with a tender, swollen joint. Carefully palpate where the maximally tender spots are, because this may help you later classify the fracture pattern. In particular, note whether there is tenderness medially, laterally, anteriorly, posteriorly, or in a combination of locations. Ankle injuries are rarely all bony; usually a combination of structures are damaged, so that a fracture may exist laterally with a pure ligamentous injury medially. The presence of tenderness medially may be your best clue that a medial component is present. Furthermore, injury on more than one side of the ankle has dramatic importance for treatment, because medial and lateral damage often produces enough ankle instability that prolonged immobilization, or more often, surgical intervention is required.

Palpate the entire leg when examining the patient, including the fibular border all the way to the knee. A Maisonneuve-type fracture, which is an unstable pattern, is a high fibular fracture, sometimes with no other radiographic abnormality (Fig. 5–2). Nonetheless, the medial side of the ankle is disrupted (deltoid ligament failure) and the lateral side is also incompetent because of failure of the syndesmotic ligaments. The fibula breaks where the injuring force exits the leg, often proxi-

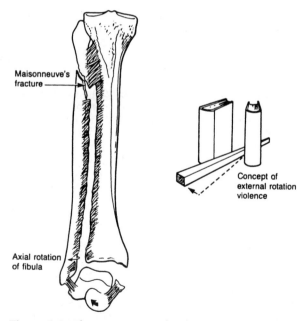

Figure 5–2. The Maisonneuve fracture. Note that external rotation causes a ligamentous injury at the ankle, which extends proximally and produces a high fibular fracture. (From Rockwood, CA, Jr., Green, DP, and Bucholz, RW [eds]: Fractures in Adults, ed 3. JB Lippincott, Philadelphia, 1991, p 1985, with permission.)

mally near the knee. So the fibular fracture may be the only radiographic tip-off that an unstable injury is present. You may never even think of getting an x-ray of the proximal leg unless you first identify tenderness there. Do not forget to scrutinize the entire leg when first assessing these patients.

Sprain

Note also that occasionally patients demonstrate severe swelling and pain and yet only have what amounts to a severe sprain. The diagnosis of sprain, however, is one of exclusion, requiring a thoroughly negative radiographic and stability assessment. Furthermore, some ankle ligament sprains can be painful enough that cast immobilization may ultimately be the best treatment, and some sprains can produce long-term problems related to persistent ankle laxity or osteochondral fracture fragments. Do not assume that sprains are minor injuries.

Radiographic Assessment

Some basic ankle terminology helpful in understanding radiographic assessment is listed in Table 5–2. Studies have shown that a 2-mm shift in the talar alignment

Table 5–2. BASIC ANKLE TERMINOLOGY

Lateral malleolus: the part of the distal fibula that contacts the lateral talus

Medial malleolus: the portion of the distal tibia that cups the medial talus (The talus is in effect cupped by the lateral and medial malleoli, which hold the talus in perfect alignment.)

Mortise: the joint space that normally exists between the talar dome and the medial and lateral malleoli (should be no more than about 4 mm wide)

Widening of the mortise: shifting of the talus toward one side of the ankle or the other, owing to a fracture or ligamentous failure that allows the talus to move within the ankle mortise (Fig. 5–3) will account for dramatic imbalance of the forces across the ankle. Since normal ankle forces during ambulation can easily approach three to five times a person's body weight, the inevitable long-term consequence of imbalance at this joint is destructive, painful arthritis. Therefore, the burden to achieve anatomic alignment of the ankle mortise joint is great.

The standard radiographic views include an AP, a lateral, and a mortise view. The mortise view is obtained by taking an AP film with the leg internally rotated approximately 20 degrees (Fig. 5–4). *Any asymmetry of the mortise joint space in comparing the medial and lateral sides is diagnostic of an unstable ankle injury.* Do not forget to obtain additional films of the entire leg if clinical examination suggests a proximal fibular injury.

Fracture Classification

No fracture classification system strikes more fear in the hearts of orthopaedic house staff than the Lauge-Hansen classification system for ankle fractures. This

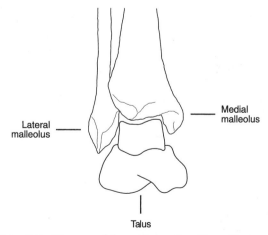

Figure 5–3. Diagram of the ankle mortise. (From Starkey, C, and Ryan, J: Evaluation of Orthopedic and Athletic Injuries. FA Davis, Philadelphia, 1997, p 87, with permission.)

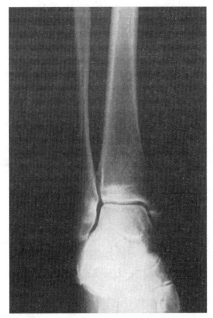

Figure 5–4. Radiograph of the normal ankle mortise (mortise projection). Note that the space between the talus and the fibula and tibia is constant. (From Donatelli, RA: The Biomechanics of the Foot and Ankle, ed 2. FA Davis, Philadelphia, 1996, p 162, with permission.)

system is moderately complicated, and most residents and medical students believe they must memorize every nuance. In actuality, very few people can wax eloquent about this system without looking at a little notecard summarizing it. In its broad presentation, the system is useful and widely popular because it proposes a logical explanation of how ankle fractures occur, and also provides a well-accepted way of quickly describing common injury patterns. Lauge-Hansen is not the only classification system, and you should be familiar with both the Lauge-Hansen system and the Danis-Weber system as proposed by the AO group from Switzerland.

The *Lauge-Hansen classification* postulates that the injury forces travel around the ankle like a circle. The position of the foot at the time of injury and the direction of the deforming force will create specific patterns of disruption. Four general locations of bone and ligamentous structures are designated: anterior, posterior, medial, and lateral. Therefore, an SER-4 injury refers to the foot that is supinated at the time of injury (weight bearing along the lateral border) and then sustains an external rotation force. Injury proceeds through all four zones (designated by the 4). Because supination is the starting position, the anterior structures are tight and represent the starting point. Therefore, the anterior talofibular ligaments rupture, then the fibula breaks, then the posterior malleolus (or posterior lip of the tibia) fails, and lastly the medial malleolus (or equivalently the deltoid ligament) breaks. The full Lauge-Hansen system is charted in Table 5–3.

The *Danis-Weber classification* is simpler in that it classifies all fracture patterns into three basic groups: A, B, and C. Table 5–4 presents an expanded Danis-Weber classification.

- Type A—fibular fracture below the syndesmotic ligaments (part of the prime stabilizers of the mortise relationship); usually stable
- Type B—fibular fracture at the level of the syndesmosis, possibly resulting in an unstable mortise
- Type C—fibular fracture clearly proximal to the syndesmotic complex, resulting in an unstable situation

Whichever classification system you become comfortable with, you should be able to broadly classify those ankle fracture patterns that are unstable.

Operative versus Nonoperative Treatment

In general, fractures of both malleoli require operative fixation because the talus can easily shift and cast immobilization will be difficult at best. Two trickier diagnostic situations are common:

1. The fibula is broken but the medial injury is purely ligamentous (deltoid ligament), so that initial x-rays may suggest only a lateral-sided injury and that the ankle may be stable. This is where your physical

Table 5-3. LAUGE-HANSEN CLASSIFICATION SYSTEM FOR ANKLE FRACTURES

Lauge-Hansen Type	Fracture Stages (in order of occurrence)
Supination-Adduction (SA)	1. Avulsion fracture (transverse) of fibula below joint level (or tear of lateral collateral ligaments) 2. Vertical fracture of medial malleolus
Supination-External Rotation (SER)	1. Tear of anterior tibiofibular ligament 2. Spiral oblique fracture of distal fibula 3. Fracture of posterior malleolus (or tear of posterior tibiofibular ligament) 4. Fracture (usually transverse) of medial malleolus (or tear of deltoid ligament)
Pronation-Abduction (PA)	1. Fracture (usually transverse) of medial malleolus (or tear of deltoid ligament) 2. Tear of syndesmotic ligaments 3. Short oblique fracture of fibula above ankle joint
Pronation-External Rotation (PER)	1. Fracture (usually transverse) of medial malleolus (or tear of deltoid ligament) 2. Tear of anterior tibiofibular ligament 3. Short oblique fracture of fibula above ankle joint 4. Tear of posterior tibiofibular ligament (or avulsion fracture of posterolateral tibia)
Pronation-Dorsiflexion	1. Fracture of medial malleolus 2. Fracture of anterior lip of tibia 3. Fibula fracture above level of ankle joint 4. Transverse fracture of posterior tibia

Table 5-4. DANIS-WEBER (AO) CLASSIFICATION OF ANKLE FRACTURES

Fracture Type	Fracture Description	Fracture Sub-Types
A	Fibula fracture below the syndesmosis	A1. Isolated fibula fracture A2. Fibula fracture with medial malleolus fracture A3. Fibula fracture with a posteromedial tibia fracture
B	Fibula fracture at the level of the syndesmosis	B1. Isolated fibula fracture B2. Fibula fracture with a medial injury (malleolus fracture or ligament tear) B3. Fibula fracture with a medial injury and a posterolateral tibia fracture
C	Fibula fracture above the syndesmosis	C1. Simple diaphyseal fibula fracture C2. Complex diaphyseal fibula fracture C3. Proximal fracture of the fibula

exam will save you, because you should be able to document that the patient is tender and swollen medially.

2. The Maisonneuve fracture, in which the medial side is injured low (medial malleolus fracture or deltoid rupture) but the lateral injury is represented by a high fibular fracture, is often underestimated (see Fig. 5–2).

If the ankle films do not clearly show a shift in the mortise, you may be fooled into thinking the patient has a stable, medial-side-only injury. Again, the physical exam will help, because you should have detected the patient's proximal fibular tenderness and then ordered full-length films and identified the lateral-side injury that characterizes an unstable situation.

In general, when the talus is stable in the mortise, operation is not necessary. Cast immobilization will be adequate to allow the injury, which is most often an isolated fibular fracture, to heal.

Initial Care in the Emergency Room

Some ankle fractures are so unstable that the talus will literally be severely subluxed or dislocated (usually posteriorly). The skin tension in these injuries is tremendous and is one reason why you should immediately realign the foot. This can be easily accomplished by pulling upward on the patient's big toe. In fact, the big toe tends to be a universal handle by which the most common fracture patterns can be provisionally reduced or improved. Let the patient's thigh externally rotate as they lie on the cart. The knee should be bent about 60 degrees. Then have an assistant support the leg by holding the great toe from above, and the ankle will experience traction, modest plantar flexion, and internal rotation. Apply your cast or splint in this position; you will be surprised at how much improved the mortise position may look.

Short-leg Splint

If the ankle has sustained injury primarily to only one side, and therefore represents a stable injury, a short-leg splint or cast will suffice. Often a definitive cast can be applied unless you anticipate unusual swelling. If a cast is applied, it is prudent to at least split it lengthwise to accommodate for swelling within the first 24 hours. Even if the injury's biomechanics would allow for weight bearing, it is a good idea to give the patient crutches (or a walker for elderly victims) and encourage keeping weight off the leg until follow-up in the office with the attending orthopaedic surgeon.

Long-leg Splint

Unstable ankle fractures require more extensive splinting, specifically a rigid device that runs proximal to the knee. This better prevents rotation at the ankle and is necessary to properly protect the ankle in unstable situations. Even if you know the patient will be going to surgery in a few hours, it is appropriate to apply a long-leg posterior mold to safely protect the ankle. In an unstable fracture situation, the weight of the foot can cause the ankle to twist or become dramatically deformed and threaten the skin and neurovascular structures crossing the joint. Painting the skin with iodine soap is also a good idea to anticipate any possible blister formation if surgery is unexpectedly delayed. Experience would suggest that you should place any fracture in the definitive protective splint in the ER, because sometimes surgery will be postponed or the patient transferred to another institution. In these situations, you have protected the patient's ankle and skin and have not allowed a delay in treatment to be compounded by a neurovascular or soft-tissue disaster.

Ankle Dorsiflexion

As a final note about cast application, for any long period of immobilization, it is best to have the ankle dorsiflexed. The talus has an asymmetrical shape in its anterior-posterior direction in that the bone is wider anteriorly. If the ankle is left in plantar flexion, it allows the mortise over time to contract and will later contribute to difficulty in regaining ankle motion in dorsiflexion. If the talus is held up in a dorsiflexed ankle, however, the mortise is kept from narrowing and ankle motion is easier to recover during rehabilitation. Forcing the ankle into dorsiflexion is not a major issue in the initial treatment because it may put more pressure on the soft tissues and typically causes more pain for the patient. Following surgical intervention or at the first office cast change, however, you may notice that most attending physicians will make a point of replacing the cast or splint with the foot dorsiflexed.

TALUS FRACTURES

Fractures of the talus occur from an axial load with the foot plantar-flexed. Patients complain of a tender, swollen foot or ankle. The physical exam may not demonstrate dramatic abnormalities except a swollen ankle and diffuse tenderness.

Radiographic assessment starts with AP and lateral plain x-rays and usually is supplemented with a CT scan. The talar neck is the most common location of fracture, and the *Hawkins system* is the most accepted way of classifying these fractures.

- Type I—Nondisplaced vertical neck fractures
- Type II—Displaced fractures that involve subluxation from the subtalar joint alone
- Type III—Displaced fractures that involve subluxation from the subtalar and ankle joint together
- Type IV—Displaced fractures that involve subluxation from the subtalar, ankle, and talonavicular joints

Because the talus communicates with the ankle joint as well as the midfoot articulations, most fractures require anatomic alignment. Furthermore, the bone is at risk of developing osteonecrosis because the talar blood supply can be interrupted by a displaced fracture. Consequently, precise assessment of fracture alignment and immediate reduction and fixation of certain displaced fractures may improve the overall outcome.

Any displacement of more than 2 mm or any joint subluxation must be corrected through operative fixation of the fracture. Typical internal fixation involves several screws and possibly bone graft. Even with nondisplaced fractures that are treated in a cast, patients usually must remain non–weight bearing for several months until it is clear that the fracture has healed.

The development of osteonecrosis of the talus correlates with the severity of injury. Usually at about 6 weeks postinjury, there is some healing of the fracture. This may be manifested on x-ray by the decreased bone density in the talar dome (the healing process actually causes bone to be initially reabsorbed). The *Hawkins sign* refers to the absence of this decrease in bone density at 6 weeks after injury and is a sign of early osteonecrosis. Painful arthritis of ankle or subtalar joint can be a result of osteonecrosis, although in one study, two-thirds of the patients who developed osteonecrosis after fracture seemed to have a satisfactory clinical outcome anyway.

CALCANEUS FRACTURES

Fractures of the calcaneus are caused by a sudden impact to the hindfoot. Falls, therefore, comprise the most common mechanism. It is surprising how much damage can be done from what seems like a short falling distance. Jumping off a wall or falling from a ladder are common scenarios.

Clinical Presentation

Patients with calcaneal fractures present with a widened hindfoot and severe pain and swelling. These fractures can produce massive swelling and are notoriously associated with compartment syndrome of the foot. Even when the fracture is minimally displaced, it is prudent to admit the patients so that appropriate monitoring of their neurovascular status can be performed during the first 24 hours.

Application of a huge, bulky, loosely wrapped dressing with a plaster splint run up to the knee will help with pain and swelling. Swelling, however, must be aggressively handled further by elevating the foot on several pillows so that with the patient partially reclining, the foot is at least as high as the heart. Be very specific in describing how the foot should be elevated when you write admission orders.

Because patients with calcaneal fractures are the victims of large axial loads, be sure to ask and inspect for other injuries. The lumber spine is a classic associated injury zone, and any complaint of back pain should be aggressively pursued with appropriate x-rays.

Radiographic Assessment

The calcaneus, like the ilium and scapula, has a peculiar shape, and it can be difficult to initially characterize injury.

The first plain film to obtain is a standard lateral view of the hindfoot. The AP view is only occasionally helpful, because other overlying bones (including part of the calcaneus) will obscure some detail.

The following two specialized views are also helpful:

1. Axial view of the heel, which will show how much the calcaneus has widened and can also demonstrate subtalar joint detail.
2. Broden's view, obtained by internally rotating the foot 45 degrees while it rests on the x-ray cassette and then directing the beam anywhere from 10 to 40 degrees cephalad. This view will highlight the posterior facet of the calcaneus, a key feature of the subtalar joint.

Almost all calcaneus fractures merit evaluation with a CT scan. Even fractures that seem to be nondisplaced may actually have subtlety that can only be appreciated with sophisticated imaging techniques. The best way to obtain the CT scan is by imaging the calcaneus in two planes perpendicular to each other, with one parallel to the posterior facet. Write these details down directly on the CT scan request form, and talk to the radiology technician yourself to make sure the scan is performed properly.

Calcaneal fractures have been classified as either "tongue" or "joint depression" type, depending on the secondary fracture line (Fig. 5–5). The primary fracture line, which is present in both types of intra-articular calcaneus fractures, divides the calcaneus body into anteromedial and posterolateral pieces (Fig. 5–6). Two radiographic measurements that are commonly mentioned include Böhler's angle and Gissane's angle, illustrated in Figure 5–7.

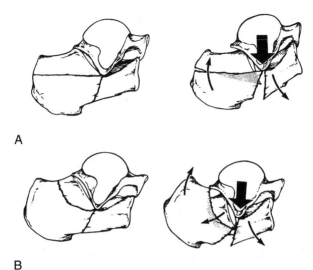

A

B

Figure 5–5. *(A)* The secondary fracture line for the "tongue" type of calcaneus fracture. *(B)* The secondary fracture line that characterizes the "joint depression" type of calcaneus fracture. (From Rockwood, CA, Jr., Green, DP, and Bucholz, RW [eds]: Fractures in Adults, ed 3. JB Lippincott, Philadelphia, 1991, pp 2117-2118, with permission.)

Treatment Considerations

Calcaneal fractures have a legacy of poor results. They account for a long period of disability because patients cannot walk satisfactorily until the fracture heals. The crushing nature of most injuries produces a widened heel and altered joint mechanics that accounts for long-term pain and problems with footwear. It is not uncommon for patients to sustain bilateral calcaneal fractures and subsequently be out of work for a year after their injury.

Closed management of calcaneal fractures has been the traditional approach, although within the past 10 years, open surgical methods have gained more popularity. *The goal of treatment is to narrow the heel, restore the height of the calcaneus, and anatomically realign the subtalar contact surfaces, especially the posterior facet.*

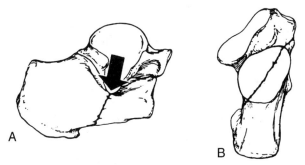

Figure 5–6. *(A)* Lateral and *(B)* anteroposterior views of the primary fracture line that commonly occurs in intra-articular calcaneus fractures. Note that two main fragments are produced: anteromedial and posterolateral. (From Rockwood, CA, Jr., Green, DP, and Bucholz, RW [eds]: Fractures in Adults, ed 3. JB Lippincott, Philadelphia, 1991, p 2116, with permission.)

Operative care is probably the best way that posterior facet damage can be reliably improved.

If surgery is undertaken, it is delayed until massive swelling of the foot has improved. Operative intervention, then, is routinely delayed for 7 to 10 days. This allows time for appropriate imaging to be obtained and helps avoid the catastrophe of surgical wound compli-

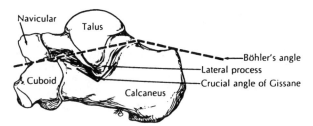

Figure 5–7. Lateral representation of the normal calcaneus, highlighting Böhler's angle (normally measuring between 25 and 40 degrees) and Gissane's angle. (From Rockwood, CA, Jr., Green, DP, and Bucholz, RW [eds]: Fractures in Adults, ed 3. JB Lippincott, Philadelphia, 1991, p 2104, with permission.)

cations related to swelling. The wrinkle sign refers to the presence of normal skin wrinkles in the foot and heel and is a demonstration that soft-tissue tension has diminished to near normal levels. Most surgeons will not contemplate operation until the wrinkle sign is present.

FRACTURES ABOUT THE MIDFOOT

Clinical Presentation and Treatment Considerations

The bones about the midfoot include the cuneiforms, tarsal navicular, and the cuboid. Cuneiform fractures are relatively rare and can usually be managed by immobilization with protected weight bearing until healing has occurred.

Injury to the tarsal navicular may present as a stress fracture or as an acute fracture. Intra-articular fractures that are displaced may require internal fixation to correct articular incongruity and reduce the likelihood of posttraumatic arthritis.

Cuboid crushing fracture can occur from lateral deforming forces applied to the forefoot. If severe loss of height occurs, some authors are recommending operative treatment with bone graft to restore the cuboid's overall shape. This crushing-type injury has been termed the "nutcracker" fracture.

Lisfranc's Injury

In addition to these fractures, most of which are relatively rare and are often treated nonoperatively, the critical injury of the midfoot is the Lisfranc lesion. This is a fracture-dislocation of the tarsal-metatarsal joints and, if untreated, carries a predictably poor prognosis with respect to painful arthritis.

The *mechanism of injury* is usually some sort of hyperextension at the forefoot with an applied axial load. There is a high association of other metatarsal fractures being present with Lisfranc joint injuries, so examine the entire foot carefully. In any patient with a foot injury, be careful to meticulously palpate the tarsal-metatarsal area, and if any tenderness, instability, or swelling is present, be sure to check appropriate radiographs screening for this injury pattern. It can be easy to miss a Lisfranc fracture, and again, the missed injury can have an especially poor outcome.

Radiographic assessment consists of AP, lateral, and oblique views of the midfoot. Critical x-ray landmarks are the metatarsal base alignments with the adjacent bones. For example, the second metatarsal's medial edge should line up perfectly with the medial border of the second cuneiform. The medial edge of the fourth metatarsal should line up exactly with the medial surface of the cuboid. Any widening or change in these relationships or any avulsion fractures present at the metatarsal bases must be taken as a sign of instability at this joint. Figure 5–8 shows the Lisfranc joint dislocation patterns.

Initial treatment is typically a compression bandage and splint to reduce swelling and pain. Occasionally, admission may be warranted if multiple joints are involved and the specter of compartment syndrome or

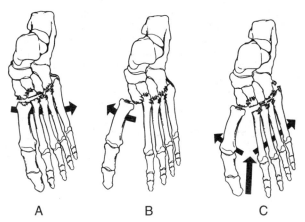

A   B   C

Figure 5–8. Three types of Lisfranc tarsometatarsal dislocations: *(A)* homolateral; *(B)* isolated; *(C)* divergent. (From Rockwood, CA, Jr., Green, DP, and Bucholz, RW [eds]: Fractures in Adults, ed 3. JB Lippincott, Philadelphia, 1991, p 2144, with permission.)

soft-tissue compromise is an issue. However, most important is the identification that an unstable Lisfranc joint is present and then treating it with definitive reduction and stabilization. Surgery can be undertaken within a few days when swelling has diminished. Meticulous realignment of the affected tarsal-metatarsal joints is often secured with multiple pins or screws.

METATARSAL AND TOE PHALANGEAL FRACTURES

Metatarsal Fractures

The most common metatarsal fracture occurs at the base of the fifth metatarsal. The mechanism of injury is typically a sudden inversion of the foot, such as occurs when the patient takes a misstep off an elevated curb. The peroneal tendon attachments produce a traction force that causes an avulsion type fracture at the fifth metatarsal base.

Even if displacement of a few millimeters is present, these "base-of-the-fifth" fractures can be treated symptomatically. It probably does not matter whether you put your patients in a walking cast, wrap them in bulky dressing and give them a hard-soled shoe, or apply an Unna boot. (An Unna boot is a roll of gauze-type bandaging impregnated with calamine lotion. It can be applied over a layer of cast padding and hardens over a day or so. It creates a semirigid, conforming foot bandage that sometimes is a nice compromise between a totally rigid cast and a nonrigid Ace bandage.) Most of these fractures heal reliably within 6 weeks, and protected weight bearing and supportive care are usually all that is necessary.

Patients who seem to be less reliable or have a low pain threshold may do better with a cast for the first 3 weeks. Sometimes the ER physician will have a specific preference for treating these common injuries, and if your orthopaedic attending physician does not care, it can be most expeditious (and politically prudent) to apply whatever treatment method the ER physician prefers.

The *Jones fracture* is a fracture through the proximal metatarsal shaft and should not be confused with the base-of-the-fifth-metatarsal fracture. The blood supply of this zone has been noted to be poor, and occasionally, the Jones fracture proceeds to a nonunion fracture unless treated with aggressive immobilization or surgical internal fixation. Initially, a proximal fifth metatarsal shaft fracture should be placed into a formal short-leg cast, and the patient instructed to remain non–weight bearing. It may be helpful to inform the patient right away that sometimes these fractures do not heal readily and occasionally require surgical care.

Most other metatarsal fractures are treated closed unless unacceptable joint incongruity, bony angulation, or rotational deformity is present. If multiple adjacent metatarsal fractures are present, surgical fixation is often required to restore forefoot stability and alignment.

Toe Fractures

Most toe fractures can be treated nonoperatively. In fact, most can be treated by simply taping the affected toe to an adjacent normal one, which will provide some immobilization. Application of a cast to immobilize a toe fracture is useless. The best method to help protect the injured toe is have the patient wear a hard-soled shoe, which facilitates weight transfer to the heel and away from the forefoot. Occasionally, a severely displaced phalangeal fracture or an articular injury justifies operative pinning.

You may be occasionally paged by a patient who is at home and states, "I stubbed my toe and it might be broken, but I don't need to have it looked at by a doctor because there's nothing you can do for it anyway, right?" Do not be fooled. You cannot safely provide medical advice without properly evaluating the patient. Sometimes a person has a severe injury that requires specific intervention. Encourage anyone who asks you about an injury to pursue appropriate assessment. This includes a physical exam by a physician and x-rays of the affected skeleton.

6

CHAPTER

Dislocations

INTRODUCTION

Definition of Terms

A *dislocation* of the joint is a displacement in which the adjacent bone contact surfaces are not touching. When describing a dislocation, the distal part is the reference point. For example, a "posterior" hip dislocation means that the femoral head is posterior to the acetabulum. An "anterior" hip dislocation means that the femoral head is anterior to the acetabulum.

Joint dislocations represent orthopaedic emergencies. *Reduction* of the dislocation, or restoration of joint congruity, should be undertaken as soon as possible not only to relieve the patient's dramatic discomfort, but also to restore normal joint stability. As with grossly unstable fractures, the soft-tissue envelope surrounding a dislocated joint bears the load of holding the extremity in place, and the nerves and blood vessels traveling through this zone can be stretched or torn. Patients demonstrate significant anxiety when moving the affected extremity and often guard the injured joint against any motion or stress. Occasionally, an acutely dislocated joint is only mildly uncomfortable if it is held completely still. However, patients still note that "something feels terribly out of place" and demonstrate great apprehension.

Subluxation of the joint means that the articular surfaces have moved out of alignment but not to the point of dislocation. Subluxations also should be reduced immediately, especially if they are dramatic. The more profound implication of a subluxation, like a complete dislocation, is that significant soft-tissue damage has occurred and the joint is unstable.

Initial Assessment

In the past, it may have been more common to treat some dislocated joints immediately "at the scene." Trainers have been known to reduce a dislocated shoulder on the football field by yanking on the arm suddenly, after which the player jumps up and runs back to the bench. However, this is probably not the best way to manage these injuries for the following two reasons:

1. It is difficult to know how to reduce a dislocated joint without knowing exactly which way the bones are malaligned. For example, the maneuver to reduce an anterior shoulder dislocation is significantly different from that used to reduce a posterior shoulder dislocation. Repeatedly struggling to reduce a joint can inflict more trauma to the extremity (and more pain and anxiety to the patient). A nerve or artery may not be pathologically stretched until the misguided treater overmanipulates the arm.
2. Appropriate x-rays of the affected joint must be obtained to look for associated fractures. For example, if fractures are later found at the margin of the joint, how does one know that the fracture occurred from the injury and not from the reduction attempt? Furthermore, fracture fragments may be trapped within the joint and physically block reduction. In some situations, an associated fracture may be the more serious injury (such as a posterior acetabular-wall fracture from a hip dislocation) and may constitute the key factor that determines treatment approach, recovery program, and outcome.

For these reasons, it is safe practice to obtain at least two orthogonal (90 degrees to each other) x-rays before treating a dislocation to determine the presence of fracture as well as the exact direction of dislocation. Keep in mind that *a single x-ray is inadequate;* for example, a posterior hip dislocation may look like a normal joint on the anteroposterior (AP) radiograph, whereas the lateral view will clearly show the problem.

Reduction in the Emergency Room

Most dislocations can be reduced in the emergency room (ER) setting with the help of sedation and anesthesia.

Sedation

The most common difficulty arises from not sedating the patient enough. Even if the patient is small and you have a body builder's physique, the muscles surrounding the joint maintain a terrific mechanical advantage over the joint's position compared with your hands. Furthermore, the harder you pull, the more pain and spasm you will create, and the patient's muscles will fight back and win. However, if the patient is properly sedated, anxiety and muscle spasm can be decreased and a quick, directed manipulation of the joint can often easily pop it back in place.

The ER staff handles a great number of dislocations without consulting the orthopaedic surgery service. However, in those cases where the staff needs help, it is often just a matter of sedating the patient more thoroughly to allow a successful reduction maneuver. It is not the size of the treating physician, but rather the size of the sedative dose that often achieves success. As always when sedating patients, appropriate monitoring (at least pulse oximetry and blood pressure measurements) and respiratory support equipment must be available. *Never* sedate anyone unless you are certain that you or personnel immediately around you can resuscitate the patient.

Anesthesia

Adequate anesthesia is also important because it allows the reduction maneuver to be performed with less force. This reduces the likelihood that you will add trauma to the joint or displace fractures while attempting to correct the dislocation.

Chronic Dislocation

It is important to establish a history of acute trauma in patients with dislocations. Occasionally, an elderly patient in distress arrives in the ER from a nursing home. No history is available and the patient cannot provide one. X-rays show a dislocated shoulder, and an hour is spent fruitlessly tugging on the arm in every possible direction. Then a relative shows up and declares that "mother dislocated that shoulder 9 years ago and it's never been in place!"

Dislocated joints that have been out of place for more than a few days may need open surgery to reduce them. Major joints that have been dislocated for more than a few weeks usually require major salvage reconstruction procedures (such as arthroplasty) to address the problem. In some situations of severely diminished function or mental status, long-standing dislocations are best left alone. Therefore, establish the exact history before manipulating the patient, especially in cases in which patient communication may be compromised.

STERNOCLAVICULAR JOINT

Clinical Presentation

Sternoclavicular joint dislocations come in two varieties: anterior and posterior.

- *Anterior dislocations* are the most common. The medial end of the clavicle moves out of contact with the sternum, and patients present with painful swelling on the affected side of their sternum. These dislocations can result from a fall in which the shoulder is impacted and forces the clavicle forward.
- *Posterior dislocations* occur from a direct blow to the chest or clavicle, as when a football player is struck directly in the chest by an outstretched arm.

It can be very difficult to identify the problem on plain x-rays because the ribs and spine are superimposed over the pathology. In addition to an AP chest x-ray, radiographic views of the sternoclavicular joint in which the beam is angled 40 degrees cephalad may be helpful. However, the surest way to assess the injury is by computed tomography (CT) scan.

In patients who are younger than 25 years old, sterno-clavicular joint dislocation often involves a growth-plate fracture (Salter type I or II; see Chapter 7) in which a small fracture fragment is avulsed off the medial clavicle.

Treatment

Treatment of sternoclavicular joint dislocation is typically nonoperative. A careful attempt at closed reduction is merited at least once, although reduction usually cannot be maintained.

Anterior dislocations that remain unreduced produce very little functional or mechanical impairment. Patients demonstrate some prominence at the affected joint, but unless pain or weakness persist after healing of the soft tissues (rarely), no other intervention is warranted.

Posterior dislocations may be more serious because they can cause compression of important structures that lie behind the clavicle, such as the trachea, esophagus, or great vessels. Compression of these structures is the main reason why a posterior sternoclavicular dislocation would require reduction.

Reduction of anterior and posterior sternoclavicular dislocations can occasionally be achieved by gently manipulating the shoulder or clavicle directly. Do not push the clavicle inward too hard or perform any dramatic maneuvers. In the case of a posterior dislocation that must be reduced owing to compression of chest wall structures, closed reduction must sometimes be accomplished in an operating room setting. With the patient prepped and under general anesthesia, the clavicle can be purchased with a towel clip–type clamp and pulled forward.

A CT scan can be of critical importance in identifying compromise of adjacent anatomy. Watch for the patient with a posterior sternoclavicular dislocation who complains of difficulty swallowing! Potential compression of the subclavian vessels increases the value of performing a careful neurovascular exam of the upper extremities.

Prognosis

It often takes 3 to 6 weeks for soft tissues around the joint to heal; patients may find use of a sling for the first 3 weeks helpful. Sporting activities should be limited for at least 3 to 4 months after injury.

ACROMIOCLAVICULAR JOINT

Dislocation of the distal clavicle from the acromion is termed a "shoulder separation." The clavicle is normally held in position to the acromion by two sets of ligaments (Fig. 6–1): the acromioclavicular (AC) ligaments (which surround the AC joint) and the coracoclavicular (CC) ligaments (which hold the clavicle vertically stable by anchoring the distal shaft to the coracoid process of the scapula).

Acromioclavicular joint separations are graded in severity as follows, depending on the instability of the distal clavicle.

- Type I—AC joint ligaments are stretched.
- Type II—AC ligaments are torn completely, and the distal clavicle is subluxed superiorly.

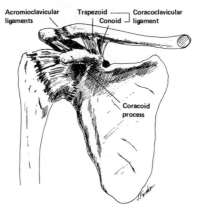

Figure 6–1. The acromioclavicular ligaments and coracoclavicular ligaments. (From Norkin, CC, and Levangie, PK: Joint Structure and Function: A Comprehensive Analysis. FA Davis, Philadelphia, 1983, p 163, with permission.)

- Type III—Both the AC ligaments and the CC ligaments are torn, and complete superior dislocation of the clavicle occurs.
- Type IV—Complete clavicle dislocation results in severe displacement posteriorly.
- Type V—Complete clavicle dislocation results in severe displacement superiorly.
- Type VI—Complete clavicle dislocation results in severe displacement inferiorly.

Clinical Presentation

The most common mechanism of injury is a fall onto the lateral aspect of the shoulder, classically off a motorcycle or a bicycle. Patients present with acute tenderness and swelling over the AC joint. The brachial plexus can be easily stretched in this scenario, especially if the patient's head and shoulder undergo traction as the upper torso hits the pavement.

Documentation of the injured extremity's neurovascular status is particularly important. AP x-rays demonstrate clavicle subluxation, if present. Sometimes obtaining comparison views of the uninjured AC joint is helpful. Radiographic assessment has traditionally also included weighted films, which are shoulder films with the patient holding a heavy weight in the injured arm. These theoretically would highlight any potential separation between the clavicle and the acromion, although weighted AC films are now not as popular as they once were. Most authors believe any significant joint subluxation will be obvious on plain films, regardless of what the patient is holding.

Treatment

Although it seems logical that any subluxation of the AC joint should be reduced and held reduced, in reality this is rarely possible. The distal clavicle cannot be reliably held in position with any external appliance, nor does it need to be. Even in type III separations, patients eventually resume pain-free function of the shoulder without any dramatic intervention. Only in cases of severe displacement, as in type IV, V, or VI injuries, do most authors agree that surgical reduction and stabilization may be a somewhat more reasonable consideration.

Prognosis

It may take many months for the AC joint to become nontender, but most patients with the type I, II, or III injuries are best served with noninvasive management. Some surgeons prefer to attempt operative fixation of the AC joint for type III separations when they occur in professional athletes. However, the complications that occur from attempted internal fixation of the AC joint are legendary, and most AC injuries can be treated with a sling and a supervised motion program that commences when initial tenderness subsides after a few weeks. In some situations in which patients do develop persistent symptoms, such as clicking or painful weakness in throwing, specific reconstructive procedures can improve the ligamentous stability of the distal clavicle. However, these operations are reserved for patients in whom long-term symptoms develop, and they are infrequently performed during the acute recovery period.

Patients with the common type I, II, or III injuries can be informed that they will likely have some permanent residual cosmetic prominence of the AC joint, that their tenderness will gradually resolve over a period of 4 to 8 weeks, and that they will most likely not suffer any meaningful long-term loss of shoulder function or strength.

SHOULDER JOINT

The shoulder is one of the most common sites for a dislocation event. In contrast to the hip joint, the bony socket of the shoulder (glenoid) is relatively flat, and its stability is greatly dependent on surrounding soft-tissue structures that control position of the humeral head.

Clinical Presentation

Anterior Dislocations

Anterior dislocation is the most common variety of shoulder joint dislocation, usually caused by a trauma that accentuates external rotation and abduction of the arm. This motion forces the humeral head forward and out of contact with the glenoid (Fig. 6–2). Common scenarios include sports situations in which the patient

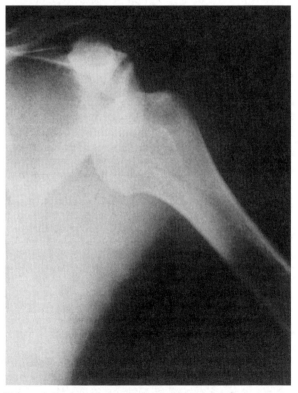

Figure 6–2. An anteroposterior radiograph of an anterior shoulder dislocation. (From Starkey, C, and Ryan, JL: Evaluation of Orthopedic and Athletic Injuries. FA Davis, Philadelphia, 1996, p 335, with permission.)

is struck on the arm while throwing or reaching over-head. Significant soft-tissue injury occurs with most dislocations, and sometimes associated cartilage ("la-bral") tears, muscle or tendon damage, or glenoid rim fractures will predispose the patient to recurrent dislo-cation episodes. A first-time dislocation results from a significant trauma, whereas recurrent dislocations due to chronic instability often occur with little provocation.

Posterior Dislocations

Posterior shoulder dislocations account for less than 5 percent of all dislocations and can be associated with violent muscle contractions that occur during seizures or electrical shock accidents. Inferior, or subglenoid, dislocation of the shoulder is referred to as *luxatio erecta*. Patients present with the humerus locked in 110 degrees or more of abduction because the humeral head is situated below the shoulder socket, usually adherent to the lateral chest wall. Patients with luxatio erecta often sustain avulsions of the rotator cuff.

Radiographic Assessment

It is essential to obtain adequate radiographic evalua-tion of the shoulder, not only to document any associ-ated fractures, but also to identify the direction of dislo-cation and verify that the shoulder has been reduced properly.

An AP view should be complemented by an axillary lateral or a scapular "Y" view to demonstrate pathology. It is very easy to miss a posterior shoulder dislocation because the AP view often appears normal, and in fact some authors propose that 50 percent of posterior shoulder dislocations are not diagnosed in the ER. (Sometimes radiology technicians attempt to shoot a transthoracic lateral x-ray because taking an axillary view requires moving the patient's arm and therefore produces pain. However, the transthoracic view is al-most impossible to read because the ribs and spine overlie the shoulder bones.) If the patient has too much pain with positioning the arm for an axillary lateral, have the technician shoot a scapular Y view, which only requires that the patient stand up. Some technicians

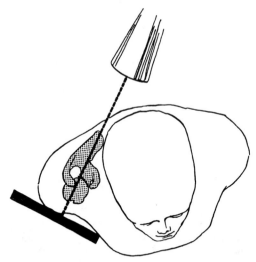

Figure 6–3. Diagram showing the technique for obtaining a "scapular Y" radiographic view of the shoulder. Note that the patient does not have to lie down or raise the arm in order for this view to be obtained. (From Rockwood, CA, Jr., Green, DP, and Bucholz, RW [eds]: Fractures in Adults, ed 3. JB Lippincott, Philadelphia, 1991, p 1064, with permission.)

will not be familiar with the scapular Y view, but it is easy to obtain, as illustrated in Figure 6–3.

As in any trauma situation, do not hesitate to accompany the patient to the radiology department and hold the extremity yourself while the technician takes the picture. In the long run, this saves time, reduces patient discomfort, and produces a useful x-ray with one exposure.

Treatment

Reduction

Reduction of a shoulder dislocation relies on moving the humeral head back toward the glenoid, so you must know which way the humerus has traveled to reach the dislocated state. Usually, gentle traction and internal or external rotation will secure reduction. Be aware that in large patients, significant sedation and muscle relaxation are prerequisites to achieving a reduction. Clearly document the reduction by repeating appropriate x-rays.

Neurovascular injury can accompany shoulder dislocation. Axillary nerve injury is reported to occur in 10 percent of anterior dislocations, so examine the patient's extremity carefully before and after manipulation. Elderly patients are at particular risk of tearing the axillary artery, which becomes less flexible with age. Be sure to check distal pulses before and after manipulation.

Hill-Sachs Lesion

Occasionally, x-rays demonstrate *Hill-Sachs lesion,* which is a trenchlike defect in the posterolateral aspect of the humeral head after an anterior dislocation. This lesion occurs during an anterior dislocation when the anterior glenoid rim digs into the back of the humeral head.

Rehabilitation

Patients should be sent home with a sling or shoulder immobilizer. The period of immobilization varies depending on the patient's age and mechanism of injury, but most patients with shoulder dislocations can start strengthening exercises and a formal rehabilitation protocol at about 3 weeks. Patients who sustain serious soft-tissue injuries about the shoulder (cartilage tears or rotator cuff disruptions) will either redislocate or rehabilitate poorly, and these situations merit additional imaging (e.g., magnetic resonance imaging [MRI]) and further work-up.

As previously noted, be certain to ask how the dislocation occurred. Sometimes noncommunicative patients (the elderly or intoxicated individuals) may present in the ER with x-rays showing a dislocation that is actually an old injury. It can be embarrassing to spend an hour fruitlessly attempting reduction only to find out later that the dislocation has been present for months or years. These situations would require major open surgery to correct the dislocation, usually hemiarthroplasty.

ELBOW JOINT

Dislocation of the elbow joint is second in frequency only to that of the shoulder.

Clinical Presentation

Most patients are either children or young adults. The mechanism for dislocation is typically a hyperextension injury, and most elbow dislocations are posterior, in which the ulna is displaced behind the distal humerus (Fig. 6–4). A varus or valgus force at the time of injury can produce associated trauma, such as fracture of the radial head or ulnar nerve injury.

Initial x-rays include AP and lateral views. Reduction is often easily accomplished under IV sedation in the ER setting. Study the x-rays carefully to assess the posi-

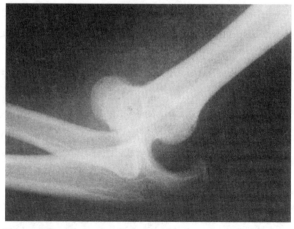

Figure 6–4. A lateral radiograph of a posterior elbow dislocation. (From Starkey, C, and Ryan, JL: Evaluation of Orthopedic and Athletic Injuries. FA Davis, Philadelphia, 1996, p 393, with permission.)

tion of the ulna relative to the humerus. To achieve reduction, (1) correct any medial or lateral displacement of the ulna, and (2) push the ulna back into the olecranon fossa by placing your thumb behind the olecranon process and pressing forward.

Associated Injuries

It is crucial to assess patients with elbow joint dislocations for associated elbow injuries. Document the neurovascular status of the arm before and after reduction, because the ulnar nerve can easily suffer a traction injury during dislocation. Also assess the x-rays carefully for radial head fractures, coronoid process fractures, or avulsions of the epicondyles. These fractures represent a more complex injury pattern and may portend elbow instability problems. In children, the medial epicondyle can become entrapped within the elbow joint and block reduction. Sometimes manipulation of the forearm in rotation can unlock this fragment and allow reduction to be accomplished. In any event, be certain that your reduction films actually show a concentrically reduced elbow and that there are no interposed bony fragments in the joint space.

Treatment

For simple elbow dislocations, the most common long-term problem is loss of motion due to prolonged immobilization. Instability is more frequently a problem if collateral ligament disruptions are present in combination with a significant radial head or proximal ulnar fracture.

For simple posterior dislocations, splint the reduced elbow in 90 degrees of flexion and give the patient a sling. Follow-up should be within 7 to 10 days, at which time the splint can be discarded and the patient can begin an active motion program.

Some adult patients may never completely regain full extension and flexion of the elbow owing to scarring of their capsule, and they should be informed of this from the start. However, with an early active motion program, most uncomplicated elbow dislocations can be rehabilitated to a near-normal functional result.

Passive stretching of the elbow should be performed later in the rehabilitation protocol, because early aggressive stretching can produce repeated bleeding in the muscles around the joint and may predispose the patient to developing heterotopic ossification.

WRIST JOINT

Dislocation of the wrist bones from the radius actually almost never occurs because the ligaments that bind the scaphoid and lunate to the radius are so stout. What does happen in cases of extreme wrist hyperextension (e.g., falling off a motorcycle) is that the weakest zone of the volar ligaments fails. This zone is between the capitate and lunate bones and can produce what is called a *perilunate dislocation*. The round head of the capitate travels dorsal to the crescentic socket of the lunate. Because the capitate and lunate occupy the distal and proximal carpal rows, respectively, other parts of these two carpal rows also must fail for this dislocation to occur. Therefore, either the ligaments around the lunate rupture (e.g., the scapholunate ligament) or the scaphoid, radial styloid, or triquetrum fractures. The injury then assumes a name that includes whatever associated fracture occurs (e.g., trans-scaphoid perilunate dislocation, Fig. 6–5).

Clinical Presentation

Because so much ligamentous or bony damage is associated with perilunate dislocations, they are typically highly unstable and dramatically severe injuries. Even so, these dislocations are notoriously easy to misdiagnose because the AP x-ray often looks "almost" normal. Sometimes the only finding on the AP film will be a slightly peculiar appearance of the lunate and capitate joint space. The lateral film, however, is pathognomonic, demonstrating the spherical capitate head sitting on top of the lunate instead of within the lunate fossa.

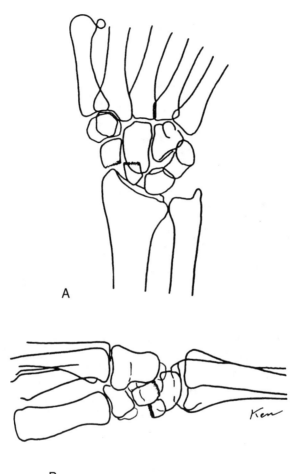

B

Figure 6–5. *(A)* Anteroposterior view of a trans-scaphoid peri-lunate dislocation. *(B)* Lateral view of the trans-scaphoid peri-lunate dislocation. This projection highlights the dorsal dis-placement of the capitate relative to the lunate. (From Tsuge, K: Comprehensive Atlas of Hand Surgery. Nankodo Publish-ing, Tokyo, 1989, pp 203 and 204.)

Although these injuries can be purely ligamentous, study the films carefully for fractures of the radius, scaphoid, triquetrum, and any other carpal bones.

Treatment

Reduction of the wrist can be accomplished by hyperextending the wrist and then gently pushing the capitate head volarly. If reduction cannot be easily accomplished in the ER, these injuries should be promptly reduced under formal anesthesia in an operating room. Sometimes the injury pattern is so complex that the exact nature of associated fractures cannot be determined until fluoroscopic examination is performed with the patient under a general anesthetic.

Because of the massive soft-tissue injury that occurs with perilunate dislocation, patients usually sustain significant permanent motion loss of the wrist even with prompt reduction and aggressive management. The most important issue to address initially is simply not missing the diagnosis. Study the lateral wrist x-ray carefully.

Other types of carpal bone dislocations can occur, such as a pure lunate dislocation, but these are extremely rare.

JOINTS IN THE HAND

Metacarpophalangeal Joint

Metacarpophalangeal (MCP) joint dislocations are most frequently dorsal. There are two types of MCP joint dislocation: simple and complex.

- *Simple (reducible) MCP dislocations* are characterized by marked deformity about the joint because the proximal phalanx is perched on the dorsal rim of the metacarpal, and this appears as a hyperextension deformity. Reduction can be accomplished by gently pushing the proximal phalanx volarly while maintaining hyperextension. The volar plate is typically detached from its proximal insertion, and aggressive longitudinal traction can entrap the volar plate between the proximal phalanx and metacarpal head, thereby converting the simple dislocation into a complex one.

- *Complex MCP joint dislocations* can be problematic. This term refers to a physical block to reduction, commonly due to entrapment of the volar plate within the affected joint (Fig. 6–6). The hallmark of the complex or irreducible dislocation is that it cannot be reduced without surgically removing the block to reduction. Furthermore, the metacarpal head of the index finger can become entangled between the lumbrical (radially) and flexor tendons (ulnarly), so that traction on the digit will actually tighten these structures like a noose around the metacarpal neck. A complex MCP dislocation will appear less deformed. Although the proximal phalanx is overriding the metacarpal head, the axes of the two bones are parallel and the digit just looks swollen without any severe angulatory deformity. Note that a telltale sign of irreducibility is dimpling of the palmar skin near the distal palmar crease. It seems as though one should be able to easily reduce this dislocation, and many times these patients will

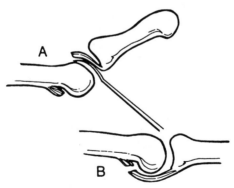

Figure 6–6. *(A)* A complex metacarpophalangeal (MCP) joint dislocation, with the volar plate blocking reduction. *(B)* If the volar plate is pulled out of the joint, reduction occurs. (From Zemel, NP: Metacarpophalangeal joint injuries in fingers. Hand Clinics 8:4, 1992. WB Saunders, Philadelphia, p 749, with permission.)

•

undergo numerous reduction attempts in the ER before orthopaedic consultation is obtained. Do not be fooled. If one or two attempts at closed reduction are not successful and there is minimal angulation present, it is probably a complex dislocation and needs operative care.

A helpful clue can be seen on the x-rays. The thumb and index finger frequently have sesamoid bones that are located within or adjacent to the volar plate. If the x-rays demonstrate the sesamoid bones within the joint space, the volar plate is surely entrapped and reduction will depend on an operative approach.

Open reduction of a complex MCP dislocation can be easily accomplished through a dorsal approach to the joint. The volar plate can be directly accessed and usually a tiny longitudinal incision in its proximal midline is enough to relax some tension on the plate and allow it to slip beneath the metacarpal head and achieve reduction of the joint.

Proximal Interphalangeal Joint

Proximal interphalangeal (PIP) joint dislocations are among the most common of hand injuries. These injuries are indigenous to the basketball court and most other ball handling sports. In most cases, the joint can be reduced with simple direct manipulation. There are two types of injuries: dorsal and volar.

- *Dorsal dislocations* are much more common than volar dislocations and involve disruption of the distal attachment of the volar plate, although the plate rarely becomes entrapped in the joint to prevent closed reduction.
- *Volar dislocations* threaten the extensor mechanism's central slip attachment to the middle phalanx. After reduction of a volar PIP dislocation, be sure that the patient can actively extend the PIP joint; if not, the central slip is probably torn and this may require operative repair. Although the volar plate becomes detached in the dorsal dislocation, it does not require repair. It seems to heal rapidly and rarely causes instability.

Occasionally, x-rays show a 1- to 3-mm fracture fragment near the base of the middle phalanx, but this is just an avulsion fracture that has occurred as a result of the volar plate injury. Despite being identified as an "articular fracture" on the radiologist's report, it is biomechanically insignificant and does not require specific intervention.

Treatment of PIP dislocations is troublesome not because of difficulty in reduction or persistence of instability, but because the PIP joint becomes remarkably stiff in a short period of time and is notoriously difficult to rehabilitate. Although instability can result from a dislocation injury, it tends to be less common than persistent stiffness. Sometimes patients are given casual advice as to how long to splint the joint or when to follow up with their doctor ("Oh, about 3 or 4 weeks..."). A *delay in supervised early mobilization can increase the likelihood of some permanent motion loss.*

Proximal interphalangeal dislocations may be splinted for 5 to 7 days to let the swelling and pain improve, but then some motion should be started. Buddy taping of the injured finger to an adjacent finger will provide some protection but also allow flexion and extension. If patients do not regain significant motion by 2 weeks, a hand therapist should be consulted to teach and supervise an aggressive stretching protocol. A little bit of education and early motion go a long way toward shortening the recovery period. Patients who first present a month after the injury without having moved the digit will probably never get all their motion back and may require 6 to 9 months of therapy to maximize their outcome.

Associated Fractures

X-rays of MCP and PIP dislocation should be scrutinized for associated fractures. Tiny avulsion fractures are usually not important, but articular fractures that make up more than 30 percent of the joint surface must be considered carefully. These fracture segments not only may require operative reduction, but also, without stabilization, will perpetuate joint instability.

HIP JOINT

Dislocation of the hip joint can represent a high-energy injury. Hip dislocations can be classified as either anterior or posterior.

The first goal should be to evaluate the patient for any other associated (and possibly life-threatening) injuries. The position of the injured extremity is often a major clue as to the direction. Posterior dislocations produce internal rotation and adduction of the leg. Anterior dislocations result in external rotation and abduction.

It is critical to reduce the dislocation promptly, because avascular necrosis of the femoral head has been related to a delay of more than 24 hours. X-rays should be scrutinized for any associated fractures of the acetabular rim or pelvis. Posterior dislocations place the sciatic nerve on stretch, so be careful to document the neurovascular status before attempting reduction.

Massive sedation may be required to reduce the hip; on occasion, general anesthesia will be necessary. Sometimes a CT scan will be helpful in making sure that there are no associated acetabular fractures and that after reduction, no significant bony fragments are interposed in the joint space.

Patients need to observe partial weight bearing on the injured limb for several weeks until their pain improves. Even in the case of an isolated dislocation that is reduced immediately, patients should be aware that they face some increased risk of posttraumatic arthritis or avascular necrosis developing over the next several years.

Dislocation of the hip joint after an arthroplasty is covered as a separate topic in Chapter 13.

KNEE JOINT

Dislocation of the knee joint is a relatively rare but potentially catastrophic injury.

Clinical Presentation

In dislocation of the knee joint, the tibia displaces either anteriorly or posteriorly relative to the femur, usually from a high-energy trauma. Occasionally, patients describe running and getting their leg caught in a deep hole, which then locks the tibia in place while the femur continues forward. Posterior dislocations are more common than the anterior type, but in either situation, the popliteal artery is at risk.

The *popliteal artery* is fixed in a soft-tissue tunnel behind the distal femur. Just distal to the knee joint, the artery trifurcates and is also anchored firmly in place. Therefore, when the knee joint dislocates, the artery is dramatically stretched and often tears or suffers intimal damage. It is therefore crucial to assess the patient's neurovascular status and also to obtain an arteriogram of the injured leg. The arteriogram is required even if the leg appears to be well perfused, because sometimes intimal damage to the popliteal artery will not cause vascular compromise until many hours later.

Treatment

The first step is to gently reduce the knee dislocation by pushing the tibia in the appropriate direction. An arteriogram of the lower extremity should then be obtained immediately to confirm vascular integrity. The extremity should also be carefully splinted to provide support across the knee joint.

Sometimes the joint will have been reduced on the field or en route to the hospital, so you need to suspect a knee dislocation in any patient who presents with a dramatic acute instability. Typical findings are medial or lateral laxity in combination with anterior or posterior instability.

These injuries require surgical intervention because the main soft-tissue structures that support the joint are severely disrupted. This includes the anterior cruciate and posterior cruciate ligaments, the joint capsule, and the collateral ligaments. Reconstructive surgery is often performed within a few weeks of the injury.

Patellar Subluxation

Occasionally, patients claim that their knee dislocated from minor trauma or that it has dislocated many times in the past. They are probably referring to subluxation of the patella. This is entirely different from knee dislocation. Patellar subluxation, although dramatically painful and clinically deforming, can be routinely reduced with gentle thumb pressure on the kneecap. Neurovascular compromise is not usually an issue. Adolescents or young adults, particularly those with inherent ligamentous laxity, may be prone to repeat episodes. Sometimes an elective soft-tissue tightening or patellar realignment procedure is necessary. Occasionally, a piece of bone or cartilage breaks off the undersurface of the patella and requires arthroscopic inspection and treatment.

JOINTS OF THE ANKLE AND FOOT

Ankle Dislocation

Like the wrist, the ankle rarely has an isolated dislocation. The talus is firmly held in place by the shape of the distal tibia and fibula. Talar subluxation or dislocation therefore almost always involves lateral, medial, or posterior malleolar fracture. The most common presentation is for the talus to be subluxed posteriorly. This can be reduced by holding the great toe and gently lifting the leg. This action often pulls the talar dome back into the ankle mortise and also often improves alignment of the associated fractures. Definitive treatment is based upon the pattern of ankle fracture, and surgery is commonly required to restore stability by internally fixing the fractures.

Tarsal-Metatarsal Joint Dislocation

Injury to the tarsal-metatarsal joint, or Lisfranc's joint, is easy to miss and can present primarily as a subluxation or dislocation pattern. A Lisfranc fracture-dislocation can occur from midfoot hyperextension and axial load. Patients present with a tender, massively swollen midfoot.

Radiographic diagnosis of this injury requires that the exact relationships of the metatarsal bases and the tarsal bones be carefully assessed. In addition to AP and lateral films, oblique midfoot films help to show the following anatomic metatarsal relationships.

- The medial border of the second metatarsal should line up perfectly with the medial border of the second cuneiform.
- The medial border of the fourth metatarsal should be congruent with the medial border of the cuboid.

Any loss of these relationships or splaying apart of the metatarsal bases must be identified and treated. In addition, small avulsion fractures at the metatarsal bases are also clues that the tarsal-metatarsal joints have been damaged.

Untreated Lisfranc injuries are notorious for producing long-term pain and arthritis of the midfoot, so the burden of prompt recognition and treatment is great. Management involves realigning the metatarsal-tarsal relationships and often requires pinning the involved joints to ensure proper healing.

Metatarsal-Phalangeal Joint Dislocation

Dislocation of the metatarsal-phalangeal (MTP) or interdigital joints of the toes is less common than dislocation of the corresponding joints in the hand. After reduction, toe dislocations rarely produce any long-term instability or functional loss, and patients frequently are back to normal after a few weeks of protected activity.

7

CHAPTER

Pediatric Fractures

THE GROWTH PLATE

Definitions

The *physis* is the actual growth-plate area, which usually appears as a thin, radiolucent band near the end of a long bone. The *epiphysis* is that area of bone between the physis and the nearest adjacent joint. The *diaphysis* is the shaft of the long bone. The *periosteum* is the thick lining that surrounds the bone.

Growth-Plate Fractures

Fractures in the pediatric population are different from those in adults for the following reasons:

- The child's bone is still growing and injury to the physis, or growth plate, may result in abnormal subsequent development. Such injury can cause the growth plate to stop altogether or just slow down enough so that bone grows slower than usual. Slower-than-normal growth can produce deformity if part of the bone grows normally and another area is delayed, because continued longitudinal growth in this situation will result in angulation (bending) at the injury site. Delayed or arrested growth of the whole physis can result in one limb being shorter than the other (as the uninjured side continues to grow at the normal rate).

- The periosteum is extremely thick in children and accounts for the faster healing times that characterize pediatric biology.
- The thick periosteal sleeve also provides some mechanical support to the bone that accounts for slightly different fracture patterns.

Pediatric fractures that involve the growth plate can be classified according to the Salter-Harris classification system (Fig. 7–1), which is the time-honored standard in describing these injuries:

- Type I—Fracture that travels through the physis and typically does not result in any displacement of the epiphysis or that portion of the bone distal to the physis. The physis will appear as a radiolucent bar on the film, and a nondisplaced fracture through this zone will not show up.
- Type II—Similar to a type I injury except that a triangle of metaphyseal bone breaks off with the distal segment, demonstrating that the fracture line has crossed directly through a portion of the physis.
- Type III—Fracture line that travels from the joint line through the epiphysis to the physis and then exists across the physis, creating a rectangularly shaped segment of the epiphysis that is a free fragment.
- Type IV—Fracture line that travels from the joint surface through the epiphysis and continues di-

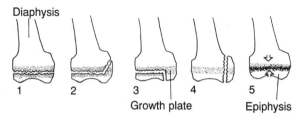

Figure 7–1. The Salter-Harris classification of growth-plate fractures. (From Singer, AJ, Burstein, JL, and Schiavone, FM: Emergency Medicine Pearls: A Practical Guide for the Efficient Resident. FA Davis, Philadelphia, 1996, p 204, with permission.)

rectly across the physis to exist somewhere proximally in metaphyseal bone.

- Type V—A crushing injury that results in significant compression (and destruction) of the epiphysis and physis.

As you may have guessed, the prognosis for subsequent growth alteration increases as the Salter-Harris category increases. For example, a Salter-Harris I injury is unlikely to produce a long-term problem, whereas a type V injury to the distal femur may result in dramatic limb-length discrepancy that requires multiple operations to correct. The age of the child at the time of injury is a major factor as well, because if the patient has a lot of growth remaining (young age at time of injury), there is a greater chance that even a small change in physeal growth will become clinically meaningful.

Treatment of displaced growth-plate fractures generally focuses on perfect realignment of the fracture pieces so that the physis has the best chance of continued development without producing deformity.

Salter I Fractures

Salter I fractures can be perplexing because the radiographs appear normal. The fracture occurs through the growth plate (which is radiolucent) but, by definition, does not produce displacement of any ossified areas (metaphysis or epiphysis). Therefore, the x-rays appear normal and diagnosis of this injury relies primarily on the physical exam of the patient. A Salter-Harris I fracture is typically a clinical diagnosis, characterized by tenderness and swelling directly over the growth plate The affected part of the extremity will be swollen and tender and possibly even a little bit unstable. In fact, the physical exam will be similar to that for a sprained joint. In children, however, the ligaments around the joint are less likely to fail than is the physis, and therefore most of these "sprain-"type presentations represent Salter I fractures. If you are careful about the physical exam, you can confirm that the patient is actually most tender directly over the bony physis and not actually at the ligaments.

Fortunately, most Salter I fractures are easy to treat because no bony displacement is present and the likelihood of future growth arrest is slim. Typically, simple immobilization in a cast will suffice.

TORUS FRACTURES

Torus fractures are injuries that represent slight buckling of the bone's cortex. They usually result from mild to moderate axial load of the bone. The force is just enough to cause the bone to "crinkle" or buckle, but not enough to grossly break into discrete pieces. This fracture pattern is characteristic of children because their bones are "rubbery" enough to fail by buckling. The adult skeleton is much more brittle (and has a thinner periosteum) so that axial load injuries usually result in distinct, separate fracture fragments.

Common locations for torus fractures include the distal radius and distal tibia, the latter of which is commonly referred to as a "toddler's fracture."

Torus fractures are not displaced, angulated, or shortened enough to require any corrective manipulation. In fact, they may be so minor that it becomes difficult to identify their presence on x-ray. It is common for parents to bring their children in for evaluation several days after the injury because there is initial doubt that an injury is present. However, the child will usually persistently favor the affected arm or leg, and after a night or two of restless sleep, the parents bring the child to the office or emergency room (ER).

Despite the benign radiographic appearance, torus fractures are legitimate bony injuries that produce bleeding, swelling, and pain. This is true even for the most minor torus injuries, which appear on x-ray only as a tiny dimple in the bone's cortical margin. It is by far the best overall plan to immobilize the affected extremity in a cast for several weeks until the bone starts to heal. It helps to explain to the parents that the cast is not truly required to hold alignment of the bone, but rather functions as a protective covering that prevents additional injury or constant aggravation of the injury site. Most children demonstrate remarkable pain relief within 1 or 2 days of being placed in a cast.

Cast immobilization in patients with torus fractures requires a little extra attention, because many infants or toddlers can (and will) remove a short-arm or short-leg cast. This is especially true in infants, because the extremity tends to be rather chubby and round, making it difficult to adequately mold the cast. Application of a long-arm or long-leg cast (with the elbow or knee bent 90 degrees) works better, because this type of cast is much more difficult for the patient to wriggle off.

GREENSTICK FRACTURES

The term "greenstick" refers to the pliable character of an immature tree branch. In contrast to adult bones, which are more likely to break completely into two or more parts, a child's diaphysis behaves like the green stick because the thick periosteum protects the cortex to some degree. A young child's bone actually bends quite a bit before breakage. When it does break (particularly in the forearm), a fair amount of cortex and periosteum are still intact, preventing the two pieces from separating. In addition to a thick periosteum, the child's bony cortex is more flexible (or "plastic"). Consequently, it can bend considerably before a gross crack develops. In fact, sometimes the bone bends enough to stay partially bent without any true fracture line occurring. This injury is referred to as a *plastic deformation* and may occasionally be severe enough that manipulation (under anesthesia) is required to improve the bone's appearance.

Reduction

Greenstick fractures can be difficult to reduce because even with significant manipulation the fracture often tends to "bounce" back to its bent position. In some situations, consideration may be given to purposely breaking the bone more completely so that a proper reduction is easier to obtain and hold. Sometimes an adjacent bone (such as the ulna) may be minimally injured, making the correction even more difficult to achieve. Note that such instances would require an operative anesthetic. From a practical standpoint, however, forcibly completing the fracture or breaking an adjacent bone is rarely necessary. Usually treatment of a greenstick fracture simply involves correction of deformity by first correcting the rotation of the forearm.

The question of which way to rotate the arm can be addressed by the "rule of thumb." This means that the patient's forearm should be rotated so that the thumb is turning toward the apex of angulation. Therefore, a volarly angulated fracture would be corrected by pronating the forearm.

FRACTURE LOCATIONS

Clavicle

Fractures of the clavicle are extremely common in the pediatric population. The indications for surgical management are almost nonexistent unless the fracture is open (rare). Despite whatever separation or angulation may be present on x-rays, simple symptomatic care is all that is required because clavicular fractures reliably heal and rarely result in any functional impairment or residual discomfort.

Communication with Parents

Perhaps the most important skill in treating pediatric clavicle fractures is communicating well with the parents. Patients are often alarmed at the radiographic appearance of the fracture site and also confused by the various sling or strap devices provided by the ER. It is important to carefully review the x-rays with the parents, pointing out that healing of this bone requires neither immobility nor direct contact between the pieces because of the thick periosteal tube that is present, but invisible on x-ray. *The amount of orthopaedic intervention required (little) may be inversely proportional to the amount of explanation and reassurance needed by the parents (a lot).*

It is also helpful to note that a large bump often develops at the fracture site, which represents the abundant callus (new bone) formation characteristic of a vigorously healing pediatric fracture. This bump may decrease in size over time as a remodeling process occurs, but this may take months (or even years) and some residual prominence may be permanent. Rarely does such a bump constitute a functional or even cosmetic problem.

Pain from a clavicle fracture in a child usually improves dramatically within 2 to 4 weeks.

Use of a Sling

A clavicle "figure-of-eight" harness or sling may provide more comfort by encouraging retraction of the shoulders, but no strapping device produces any significant improvement in bony alignment. The main purpose of such straps is to provide short-term pain relief. Therefore, whichever appliance seems to work best (and is least difficult to use) is the one to recommend. Some parents and children will find the figure-of-eight harnesses a nuisance to apply or painful owing to excess pressure on the skin. In these situations, it may be better to recommend use of a simple arm sling, which helps remind the patient (and those around him or her) that the arm is injured and is to be avoided.

Distal Humerus

Distal humeral fractures are extremely common in children, perhaps second only to clavicle fractures. Pediatric elbow injuries can be confusing because there are several growth plates in this region, and much of the bony anatomy is not radiographically apparent until the growth plates (and their associated epiphyses) ossify. Knowing the ossification sequence for these epiphyseal regions can be helpful to allow the physician to predict what a normal elbow should look like for a given child's age.

The mnemonic for ossification appearance of the elbow is "CRMTOL." This stands for *c*apitellum, *r*adial head, *m*edial epicondyle, *t*rochlea, *o*lecranon, and *l*ateral epicondyle. The corresponding ages in years for appearance of these centers are (approximately) 1, 3, 5, 7, 9, and 11, respectively. When evaluating a child's elbow for injury, it can be extremely helpful to obtain identical x-rays of the opposite (uninjured) elbow for comparison purposes.

The two most common fracture patterns are the supracondylar fracture and the lateral condylar fracture.

Supracondylar Fractures

Supracondylar fractures of the distal humerus are particularly common in the 4- to 8-year-old population because the elbow is still usually hyperextendable and the supracondylar region of the distal humerus is quite thin at this age. A fall on an outstretched arm can easily push the elbow into hyperextension resulting in a snap of the supracondylar area. This produces the most common (>95%) pattern of displacement, which is with the distal fracture segment posterior to the humeral shaft (called an extension-type supracondylar fracture). If any significant angulation is present (or any displacement), many orthopaedic surgeons prefer to reduce the fracture in the operating room and stabilize it with percutaneous pins. Truly nondisplaced supracondylar fracture can be treated with a simple long-arm cast.

Supracondylar fractures are potentially dangerous because they can be associated with early neurovascular compromise of the limb (Fig. 7–2). Traction or injury to the brachial artery may produce a forearm compartment syndrome. The sharp end of the humeral shaft can tear or puncture any of the three major nerves in the area. Injury to the median nerve is probably the most common.

Supracondylar fractures should be evaluated carefully and expeditiously. Document the motor, sensory, and vascular status of the limb and then contact your attending physician immediately. For displaced fractures, the sooner the bone is realigned, the less likely there will be a problem from severe swelling or tension on neurovascular structures. As a result, many orthopaedic surgeons prefer to treat displaced supracondylar fractures as emergencies and pin these injuries as soon as possible. Do not let the children eat anything while they wait in the ER.

Lateral Condylar Fractures

Lateral condylar fractures represent Salter IV injuries of the distal humerus. They are less likely than supracondylar fractures to cause immediate neurovascular problems. However, the long-term complications that can arise from lateral condylar injuries are numerous. This is because the injury can produce irregularities in

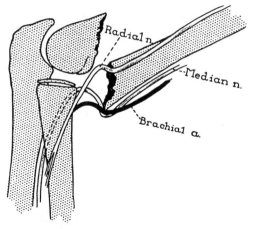

Figure 7–2. Schematic diagram of an extension-type supra-condylar humeral fracture. Note that the proximal (humeral shaft) segment can jeopardize the neurovascular bundle by producing tension over a sharp spike of bone. (From Lipscomb, PR: Vascular and neural complications in supracondylar fractures of the humerus in children. J Bone Joint Surg 37A(3):487–492, 1955.)

the growth plate, producing undergrowth or over-growth of the lateral distal humerus as the child increases in age.

The treatment of lateral condylar fractures focuses on anatomic reduction of the fracture, both because the fracture line extends to the joint surface and also because the injury crosses the growth plate (Fig. 7–3). These fractures can be classified based on displacement:

- Type I—no displacement
- Type II—up to 2 mm of displacement
- Type III—more than 2 mm of displacement

If absolutely no displacement is present, a long-arm cast may suffice for definitive care. However, for those fractures with 2 mm or more displacement, percutaneous pinning, or more commonly, open reduction, is required to perfectly reduce the fracture and decrease the probability of growth disturbance in the future.

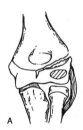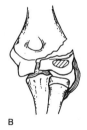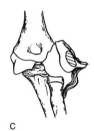

Figure 7–3. Types of lateral condyle fractures, based upon degree of displacement: *(A)* nondisplaced; *(B)* mildly displaced; *(C)* completely displaced and rotated. (From Green, NE, and Swiontkowski, MF [eds]: Skeletal Trauma in Children, ed 2. WB Saunders, Philadelphia, 1997, p 290, with permission.)

For any elbow injury, even if a long-arm cast is the definitive treatment choice, it is wise to initially immobilize the extremity with a splint or a widely split cast. Swelling in the first 72 hours can be dramatic. Therefore, whatever bandage you apply should be able to accommodate the increase in extremity diameter so that compartment syndrome or associated soft-tissue compromise is less probable.

Forearm

Shaft fractures of the radius and ulna in children ("both bone" fractures), in contrast to those fractures occurring in adults, can usually be treated nonoperatively. Although rigid internal fixation is required in adults for reliable healing, children again benefit from thick periosteum and shortened times to callus formation. Furthermore, because of the bony remodeling process that is characteristic of the growing extremity, perfect alignment is not necessary to produce an excellent outcome.

Fractures in children of the radial and ulnar shafts, or the Monteggia or Galeazzi lesions (see Chapter 4), are typically managed with closed reduction and a long-arm cast. A key element of reduction depends on rotational alignment of the forearm, with the goal of matching the distal ends of the bone to the proximal fracture segments.

As the patient's age increases, less deformity is acceptable because the effect of remodeling will be less. Remember that residual deformity in a plane of motion is better tolerated than deformity in a less mobile plane. For example, a residual forearm flexion deformity is less of a problem than a deformity of forearm radial deviation, because the former can be well compensated for with wrist motion.

Forearm shaft fractures in teenagers can be tricky because the exact age at which the fracture assumes an adult "personality" is unclear. It may become appropriate to consider operative management of displaced, unstable shaft fractures if closed reduction is difficult or has to be repeated several times.

Femoral Shaft

Femoral shaft fractures in children under the age of 10 years are usually treated nonoperatively. For infants and toddlers up to the age of 2 years, application of a hip spica cast is often the preferred initial and singular treatment. Anatomic alignment of the fracture is not necessary. In fact, because the fracture tends to stimulate overgrowth at the injury site, a loss of up to 2 cm in initial length can be desirable, because subsequent overgrowth of the femoral shaft length during healing will make up for this shortening and result in normal limb length. Application of a hip spica cast typically requires a general anesthetic.

Femoral shaft fractures that occur in the 2- to 10-year-old population are usually treated for the first few weeks with skeletal traction (Fig. 7–4). A pin is placed in the distal femur and used to hold the leg in proper length and alignment. After 2 or more weeks, enough healing may be present that the patient can be safely converted into a hip spica cast without losing significant length.

Ankle

Ankle fractures in adolescent patients can assume a confusing radiographic presentation because of involvement of the distal tibial and fibular growth plates. As

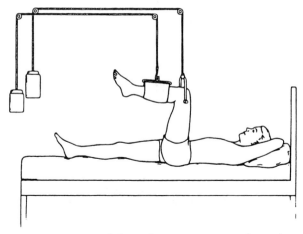

Figure 7–4. Femoral "90-90" traction, commonly used to manage femoral shaft fractures in children. (From Wolinsky, PR, and Johnson, KD: Femoral shaft fractures. In Browner, BD, Jupiter, JB, Levine, AM, and Trafton, PG [eds]: Skeletal Trauma, ed 2. WB Saunders, Philadelphia, 1997, p 1954, with permission.)

the patient approaches skeletal maturity, the distal tibial and fibular growth plates start to close in a predictable sequence, with the medial portion of the physis closing first, followed by closure of the lateral tibial physis over the next year or so.

An injury occurring during adolescence can produce a fracture through part of the distal tibial epiphysis in which the lateral portion breaks away, leaving the medial part attached to the tibia through its fused growth plate. This creates a Salter III type fracture, which is sometimes referred to as a *juvenile Tillaux lesion* (Fig. 7–5).

Severe external rotation of the adolescent ankle can produce a more complicated pattern involving two or three pieces of the lateral epiphysis with a portion of the tibial metaphysis attached. This pattern is referred to as a *triplane fracture* and again results from injury that occurs during the period when the distal tibial

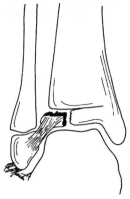

Figure 7–5. The juvenile Tillaux fracture, which is a Salter-Harris type III fracture of the distal tibial physis. This occurs in adolescents who sustain injury to their ankle when the medial portion of the distal tibial physis is fused, but the lateral portion is still open. (From Rockwood, CA, Jr., Green, DP, and Bucholz, RW [eds]: Fractures in Children, ed 2. JB Lippincott, Philadelphia, 1984, p 1023, with permission.)

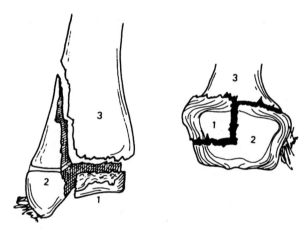

Figure 7–6. The triplane fracture. The three fragments produced by this injury are (1) the anterolateral part of the distal tibial physis; (2) the remaining physis and attached spike of tibial metaphysis; (3) the distal tibial metaphysis. A CT scan is frequently helpful in assessing this complex fracture. (From Rockwood, CA, Jr., Green, DP, and Bucholz, RW [eds]: Fractures in Children, ed 2. JB Lippincott, Philadelphia, 1984, p 1023, with permission.)

physis is partially fused (Fig. 7–6). This fracture pattern usually occurs in children between 12 and 16 years.

Any of the latter physeal ankle injuries require anatomic reduction for best results. The fracture patterns can be complicated enough that a computed tomography scan of the ankle is often ordered to clearly identify the fracture pattern and plan for reduction.

8

CHAPTER

Wounds

GENERAL PROCEDURES

You will be consulted frequently by the emergency room (ER) staff to evaluate wounds. Patients' wounds will represent a wide spectrum of injuries, ranging from simple lacerations to complete amputations. Although occasionally the general surgery service is asked to manage lacerations, anything that involves bone, nerve, tendon, or muscle is usually referred to the orthopaedic service. This means just about every type of wound is in your domain.

Some general principles can make the management of wounds much easier for you. Many times definitive care can be administered right in the ER, and knowing how to be efficient in this process can save you a great deal of time.

History

The following guidelines are important when taking the history of a patient with a laceration:

1. **Ask specifically how the laceration occurred:** If a knife or saw blade did the cutting, find out whether the blade was clean and what it is normally used to cut. For example, delicatessen-meat residue on a kitchen knife can introduce unusual bacterial flora. A lumber saw cutting plywood will undoubtedly inject wood foreign material into a wound. Lacerations

produced by glass shards may produce very small skin incisions and yet be deep puncture-type wounds that can cut a dozen tendons in one stroke. Also inquire as to how much bleeding occurred. Although patients will initially describe torrential hemorrhage, you can often distinguish from their history whether there was arterial bleeding. This information can be helpful in determining not only the likelihood of arterial injury, but also the probability of nerve injury, because many peripheral nerves travel immediately adjacent to the vessels (especially in the hand and fingers).

2. **Identify the general environment in which the injury occurred:** Wounds produced by motor boat engine blades are often complicated, not only because of their high-energy character, but also because the patient is typically immersed in lake or ocean water. Similarly, injuries due to power tools or lawn equipment also commonly involve massive contamination.

3. **Be wary when the patient is vague about the mechanism of injury:** The motivation here may relate to concealing illegal behavior, such as gang-related fighting or drug use. Individuals who are involved in drug use are more likely to have hepatitis or be HIV-positive, so be extra careful in protecting yourself when handling these wounds. Furthermore, the mechanism of injury may directly influence the treatment. For example, a 1-inch oblique laceration over the fourth metacarpal head (or just proximal to it) is highly suggestive of a human bite caused by the patient's hand striking another person's mouth. Such a laceration has particular requirements for proper treatment, as discussed later in this chapter.

4. **Document the patient's allergies:** Wound care will involve antibiotic delivery, and some patients are allergic to these drugs. Also, ask about the patient's last tetanus shot. Although the ER staff often asks about tetanus prophylaxis, get in the habit of asking the patient yourself. That way you know for sure it has been addressed.

5. **Ask the patient whether he or she has ever had a similar injury:** Aside from identifying accident-prone individuals, you may uncover a notable pat-

tern, ranging from occupational safety issues to domestic violence.

Physical Exam

Follow these guidelines when examining a patient with a laceration:

1. Look closely at the wound and record its approximate length, direction, margin character (jagged, smooth, ripping, etc.), and apparent depth. Note any obvious contamination or foreign bodies.

2. Perform a meticulous sensory and vascular exam distal to the injury. Sensibility assessment is especially important in evaluating nerves to the fingers. Test the two-point discrimination on both radial and ulnar sides of the volar fingertips. Normal static two-point discrimination is about 3 to 5 mm. Absent (or inconsistent) two-point discrimination is highly suggestive of a sensory nerve transection. Recall all the peripheral nerves traveling distal to the laceration site, and then specifically test each one for sensibility. Certain areas in the body derive sensory input from several nerves, whereas other areas of skin are almost always supplied by just one nerve. Try to find the latter areas because abnormality in these "dedicated" zones will yield the greatest specific information. In the hand, for example, sensibility at the dorsal aspect of the small finger ray is exclusively supplied by the ulnar nerve. The radial nerve is the only nerve that innervates the skin overlying the dorsal thumb and index finger web space, and median nerve sensibility can be tested by examining the volar and radial palm.

3. Perform a motor exam in the same fashion as the previous exams. Certain muscle functions can be tested to assess specific nerves. Finger abduction and adduction test the ulnar nerve, thumb extension depends on the radial nerve, and thumb abduction depends on median nerve function. A list of specific sensory and motor tests useful in examining the upper and lower extremities is noted in Appendix C.

Loss of motor function may represent either a nerve injury or perhaps a laceration of the muscle-tendon unit that accounts for motion. Sometimes both structures are cut. Remember, though, that in most situations, motor innervation is quite proximal in the extremity, whereas the discrete tendons are typically distal. Therefore, a proximal forearm laceration producing loss of wrist extension is most likely due to radial nerve injury. Loss of wrist extension from a distal (dorsal) forearm laceration is most likely due to transection of the extensor tendons. As always, a thorough understanding of anatomy will give you a tremendous advantage in diagnosing the problem.

4. Before performing the neurologic assessment, find out whether the ER staff administered local anesthetic before your arrival. Unfortunately, this practice is common because the patients are frequently in pain and quite anxious. You can be fooled into believing a nerve or tendon injury exists when in fact the extremity is merely manifesting the effects of 1 percent lidocaine.

5. Examine the entire extremity, even those areas that may initially seem remote from the skin wound. For example, the dorsal wrist and hand should be examined even in a patient who has a volar laceration. A knife blade can enter the palm, travel between the metacarpal bones, and actually cut extensor tendons without making a dorsal skin laceration. Look for swelling and discoloration. Palpate for crepitus and defects in soft-tissue continuity. A circumferential exam distal to the injury may yield surprising information.

6. It is sometimes helpful to gently pry open the wound itself and take a look. Sometimes the ends of tendons or nerves will be directly visible, confirming the injury. Seeing an open joint capsule often means a trip to the operating room. Just be careful not to probe too much unless you prepare a formal, sterile field and use sterile instruments. Also remember that being able to see bone in the base of a wound is not the equivalent of an open fracture. Many knife injuries will stop because the blade hits bone, and therefore, technically the bone is "exposed" through the wound path. If this is the extent of bone involvement,

however, it does not necessarily mandate the same care as an open fracture.

Radiographic Assessment

Get x-rays of the injured part. This is often completely neglected by the ER staff because it may seem obvious that no bones are broken. Unfortunately, not only can bones be broken by heavy blades or glass, but also the purpose of x-ray in these situations is not limited to just bone evaluation. Aside from fracture, x-rays will show foreign bodies. How do you know that the tip of the knife blade did not break off in the patient's arm?

The x-rays will also show air in soft tissues, which will help identify depth of injury penetration. Bubbly, tiny gas collections in the subcutaneous tissue may indicate gas gangrene. Careful inspection of the hand x-rays in a bar fight participant with a dorsal laceration may show a tooth mark in the metacarpal head. This indicates penetration of the joint capsule and mandates immediate surgical débridement. X-rays should be thought of as part of the physical exam.

Initial Treatment

Four issues can be addressed immediately after the history and physical exam:

1. Assess the patient's tetanus status, and, if indicated, make sure he or she receives appropriate prophylaxis in the ER. The details of tetanus prophylaxis are reviewed in Chapter 9.
2. Clean the wound of gross contaminants. Consider obtaining cultures of the wound at this point, although more and more evidence suggests that cultures obtained from acute wounds in the ER setting yield little useful information. After the wound has been cleaned, apply a temporary bandage. Even if you plan to suture the injury immediately, you will not be able to start for at least another 20 minutes, and it is good practice to cover the injury appropriately. A Betadine-soaked dressing is one good method. This way, the wound does not sit open in

the ER (the dirtiest place in the hospital), and the patient (and perhaps family) cannot stare at the bloody extremity and become more anxious.

3. Start antibiotics. It is reasonable to give the patient a dose of IV antibiotics for most wounds beyond the most superficial. Even if the patient is subsequently sent home from the ER, it is helpful to give them a single dose IV. Order the antibiotics right away and they will be running in while you finish administering care. The particular choice of antibiotics is discussed in Chapter 9.

4. Splint the injured extremity. This practice relates to the basic orthopaedic principle of resting and protecting the injured part. Even in the case of a laceration (where no fracture is present), splint application will reduce pain and anxiety. In turn, the patient will be more comfortable and calm while you go about getting the necessary equipment to repair an extensor tendon or close a wound.

Heavy Blood Loss

A caveat about blood loss from open wounds is warranted: Vigorous bleeding from an open wound is completely preventable yet produces tremendous anxiety for the patient and ER staff alike. There are two main reasons why an open wound continues to bleed vigorously beyond a few minutes:

1. The blood vessel may be *partially* cut. Partial is the key word, because a completely transected vessel will retract and shut itself down. However, a partial laceration acts to keep the vessel stretched out to length, and explosive bleeding can continue out the side wall opening. Completion of the vessel laceration will help stop the bleeding, although a better option initially is simply to apply direct pressure. In cases where the vessel merits repair, any hasty intervention in the acute setting may make surgical repair more difficult or impossible. Do not tie off vessels or cauterize anything unless you are in a surgical environment where you can see exactly what you are doing and are poised to perform definitive care. Direct pressure causes no harm and can stop bleeding from a branch of the aorta.

2. The main reason why a fresh wound continues to bleed is because the dressing is applied incorrectly. A "pressure" dressing requires pressure. Appropriate force to stop bleeding rarely derives from tape, and wrapping the bandage tight enough to immediately stop bleeding is likely to act as a tourniquet. Pressure must come from someone *holding pressure* on the wound. This can be a physician, a nurse, or even the patient. Usually a full 10 minutes of uninterrupted, firm pressure will stop any wound from continuing to bleed, unless the patient has a coagulopathy. Once bleeding has stopped, it rarely starts again unless the wound is remanipulated. A loosely wrapped, highly absorbent bandage, such as a Kerlex dressing, can actually facilitate significant blood loss from a small wound. The dressing acts as a giant absorbent suction mat that will allow even slow oozing to continue. Unless the bleeding has almost stopped and the bandage is wrapped snugly, these dressings turn into heavy, soaked mops of blood that can withdraw and hold 300 mL of blood or more. Furthermore, they get everything around them messy, and often the patient's clothing and ER linen become blood stained. Patients with a relatively small finger laceration can look as though they have been in a military battle.

Controlling Wound Hemorrhage

Finger injuries, in particular, have the potential to bleed a lot. If the digital artery is cut, blood will sometimes actually spurt across the room. Attempting to cauterize such an injury will likely vaporize the digital nerve and render the nerve irreparably damaged. Just have the patient hold direct pressure with a 2-inch-square piece of gauze under one finger and the bleeding will stop. Abrasion-type injuries at the volar finger pad also bleed vigorously. Holding a *little* pressure and then "checking" the wound every few minutes will only prolong the bleeding. Pressure must be applied continuously for more than a few minutes. Some ER staff like to apply thrombin-soaked foam material or preprepared thrombin powder to these wounds. However, this material can cost more than $100 per application, whereas simple direct pressure for 10 minutes will stop the bleeding and is free.

Some wounds may require nothing more than the steps previously noted: proper tetanus, antibiotic coverage, and a clean dressing. However, there are many instances in which some minor surgical care is required and can be administered in the ER.

The Emergency Room as Operating Room

Suturing wounds in the ER can be done efficiently if you follow a simple plan. Once the decision is made to proceed with a procedure, start by administering an anesthetic. It can take up to 10 minutes for a local anesthetic to profoundly block some parts of the body. If you give the anesthetic first, you can then spend the next few minutes setting up your equipment while the block is taking effect.

Anesthetizing the Wound with Local Anesthetic

A favorite local anesthetic agent is 1 percent lidocaine (Xylocaine). This starts to work within a minute or so and lasts 30 to 60 minutes. It can be helpful to mix the lidocaine with 0.5 percent bupivacaine (Marcaine), because the latter will prolong the block's action for more than several hours. It does take the bupivacaine more than 15 minutes to start working, so an ideal mixture is 50 percent (by volume) of 1 percent lidocaine mixed with 50 percent of 0.5 percent bupivacaine. Lidocaine's onset is quick, whereas bupivacaine will provide long duration of effect.

Local anesthetic agents are available with added epinephrine, but this is almost never used for sewing wounds. The addition of epinephrine should especially be avoided when injecting local anesthetic into the hand, because it can produce enough vasoconstriction around the fingers to produce profound digital ischemia.

After the local anesthetic is mixed and drawn up, it can be injected subcutaneously in the appropriate area with a 25-gauge needle. Sometimes it may be necessary to inject the margins of the wound that will undergo suturing.

Alternatively, some areas in the extremity can be completely anesthetized by blocking nerves proximal to the injury. For example, a very reliable way to anesthetize the finger distal to the metacarpophalangeal joint is to inject locally where the common digital nerve bifurcates in the palm. Three milliliters can be injected into the volar web space on either side of the affected digit, which will effect a "metacarpal block." Some common sites for applying blocks are noted in Appendix D.

Prepping the Patient and Your Instruments

Once the anesthetic block is in place, turn your attention to preparing the area for "surgery."

1. Unlock the patient's ER cart and move it to one side of the cubicle so that you have the most room. For example, if you are going to suture the left hand, move the cart to the far right side of the room so that you have plenty of room. Attempting to perform a procedure in cramped quarters will work against you.
2. Choose some method by which to support the limb. It may be possible to suture the lower extremities as the patient lies on the stretcher, but the upper extremities can be better positioned by placing the affected side on a Mayo stand. This position gets the forearm and hand away from the patient's side and allows you to position it just the way you want.
3. Place several large blankets underneath the affected extremity. The blankets not only prop up the field, but also serve as a large absorbent reservoir. When you prep the part and then irrigate it (often with several liters of saline), the blankets will actually absorb this much fluid and keep the patient, surgeon, and floor dry.
4. Position the patient and affected part, and then assemble the necessary instruments. Many suturing jobs can be performed with what most ERs call "a minor tray." However, these trays often have just the basic tools, and for anything slightly more involved

than a simple laceration, it might be better to get the "hand tray" or the "plastics tray." These trays usually have everything you could possibly need in the way of sterile instruments.

5. Once you put on sterile gloves, touch only what is on your sterile field and instrument tray. So it becomes a matter of efficiency that you prepare the field and collect everything you need before you finally don gloves. If you forget to get something, you will have to take your gloves off, get the item, and then reglove. Do not plan on having an ER nurse available to be your "circulating nurse" because ER nurses are too busy. It takes a minute or so to deglove and reglove if you need something, but you should try to get everything set up right once so that the procedure itself goes quickly.

6. Prep the patient's part, and then drape off a sterile field with towels. Drape off an extra large area and sterilely place your instrument tray in this zone. Some extra items that you will need include a liter of sterile saline, a sterile bowl for the saline, two scalpel blades (No. 15 blades are standard), extra sterile gloves(!), culture tubes, extra gauze bandages, a small penrose drain (handy as a tourniquet), and suture material. All these items can be amassed in your sterile field before you get started.

Use of a Tourniquet

Before beginning, decide how to achieve temporary hemostasis so you can explore the wound and perhaps suture it. In the upper extremity, you can place a blood pressure cuff on the upper arm and inflate it to 70 mm higher than the patient's systolic pressure.

Another method that is simpler and less uncomfortable is to use an Ace bandage or a small rubber penrose drain and apply a tourniquet at the level of the forearm or proximal finger. Remove all tourniquets before applying the dressing so that you confirm return of normal vascularity to the limb. Document this procedure.

Suturing the Wound

Once the anesthetic is applied, the field is prepared, your instruments are assembled, and a tourniquet is applied, you can put your gloves (and mask) on and start the procedure. The management specifics for certain wounds are noted below, but in general, use the following sequence.

1. Explore the wound to note injured structures and look for any retained foreign bodies. You may need to extend the wound proximally and distally up to an inch in each direction to completely assess the injury.
2. Once the full extent of injury is known, irrigate and clean the wound. Often 1 or 2 L of sterile saline will do.
3. After cleaning the area, proceed with definitive suturing. In some situations, this may include repairing a tendon (extensor side of the hand) or some other simple structural damage
4. Suture the skin (although note that in some scenarios, the skin is not to be sutured [see the following section on bite wounds]).
5. Apply a sterile dressing and provide clear follow-up instructions for the patient. The follow-up should be told to the patient as well as provided in writing. Two prescriptions are commonly provided: one for pain medication and the other for oral antibiotic coverage (enough for 5 days duration).

BITE WOUNDS

Bite injuries can be grouped into two categories: human bites and animal bites.

Human Bites

Most human bites result when the victim's hand strikes another person's mouth. Tooth penetration into the hand occurs from bar fights. In fact, these injuries are commonly referred to as "fight bites." As you might guess, the participants are commonly drunk, so presentation to the ER for treatment of the hand injury is variable. Some patients are seen the evening of the injury, and some come in a few days later.

In addition, the person with a bite is often reluctant to describe exactly how the laceration occurred. Suspect a fight bite in the case of any laceration overlying the metacarpal heads, particularly the fourth and fifth. The skin wound will appear to be proximal to the knuckle with the fingers extending. When the patient makes a fist, you see the wound line up better with the knuckle prominence.

Infection

Human bite wounds are treacherous. Saliva contains a plethora of bacteria and one in particular, *Eikenella corrodens*, is a gram-negative organism that can produce a dramatic, necrotizing infection. Neglected or undertreated human bites can easily produce a destructive osteomyelitis and even require eventual amputation of the digit as a salvage treatment for persistent infection. Deep infection from a fight bite can occur because the tooth penetrates the capsule of the metacarpophalangeal joint and introduces bacteria directly into this space. Note also that because the tooth penetrates the hand with the metacarpophalangeal joint fully flexed, when the patient extends the hand, the skin laceration and the capsular wound do not line up exactly. This malalignment tends to seal the joint closed.

In effect, the metacarpophalangeal joint becomes inoculated with a huge load of aggressive organisms and becomes an ideal culture environment. A lateral x-ray may actually show a small indentation of the metacarpal head, confirming that a tooth penetrated the joint.

Treatment

Human bite wounds must be treated very aggressively. Any evidence of joint penetration or tendon injury must be treated with immediate débridement in the operating room. The same is required for any patient who presents with evidence of pus draining from the wound.

Sending a patient home with oral antibiotics for a human bite is not advisable. For those patients who are seen very early and have a superficial laceration with no evidence of tendon or joint involvement, admission to the hospital for IV antibiotics and close observation is probably safer. Any evidence of more than just a superficial skin laceration is best treated with surgical débridement.

Human bite wounds must not be sutured closed. Closing the wound is the surest way to instigate a bad infection. Even after surgical débridement, these wounds are left open to facilitate drainage. Wound management consists of a wet-to-dry dressing, or a dry dressing changed frequently after soaking the wound to encourage drainage.

Antibiotic coverage is specialized for human bites. *E. corrodens* must be covered by penicillin or an equivalent, and coverage must also be provided to kill common skin organisms, such as *Staphylococcus aureus.* An acceptable protocol is to give the patients both penicillin and cefazolin (Kefzol; a good first-generation cephalosporin). An even better choice would be ampicillin/sulbactam (Unasyn), which represents single-agent therapy that provides good gram-negative and gram-positive coverage. The oral equivalent of Unasyn is amoxicillin/clavulanate (Augmentin).

Animal Bites

Dogs and Cats

Animal bite wounds can also result in severe infections. *Dogs and cats are the most common perpetrators of animal bites in this country.* Very often, the injured person is bitten while attempting to separate two fighting animals or comfort an injured one. Patients frequently present 1 or 2 days after the accident because they just do not think the wound is serious. Make sure the patient's tetanus shots are up to date and also inquire about the health of the animal. The animal must be appropriately immunized against rabies, for example, otherwise the bitten person may require rabies immunization shots.

Dog bite wounds tend to be open, ragged, tearing-type injuries, whereas cat bites are more like small, paired puncture wounds. Cat bites may seal over quickly and can develop into an abscess within 24 hours. Dog bites are more likely to drain themselves but typically represent higher-energy injuries. Such injuries can impart a great deal of direct trauma to the limb, including, for example, open fractures in the hand.

The bacterium characteristic of dog bites is *E. corodens* and of cat bites is a gram-negative organism called *Pasteurella multocida*. Therefore, as with human bites, gram-negative antibiotic coverage is required, and Unasyn is the preferred single agent.

Wound closure for dog and cat bites is contraindicated because open drainage is the best way to prevent abscess formation. Any evidence of advancing cellulitis mandates hospital admission for IV antibiotics. Wounds draining pus should be débrided initially in the operating room. Impress upon patients that dog and cat bites can require multiple operative débridements and can be very difficult to control.

Other Animals

Other common biting animals include raccoons and squirrels. Unfortunately, it is rare that the biting animal can be identified, and because rabies is a real threat in this population, bitten persons frequently require rabies immunizations.

FOREIGN BODIES

Immediate removal of foreign bodies is required in only a few situations:

- Anything that produces neurovascular compromise must be removed emergently.
- Foreign material that is in a joint space should be removed promptly to prevent damage to joint surfaces. Metal parts exposed to synovial fluid can leach out metal ions and potentially damage adjacent soft tissue and also result in metal ion absorption by the body.

For most foreign bodies that are buried within a wound, no immediate treatment is necessary. If you can actually see part of the foreign body sticking out of the wound, go ahead and try to remove it directly. However, if you cannot easily see the such material, attempting to dig around in the wound to find it will likely be unrewarding.

A common scenario is a child who presents with a pin or sewing needle stuck an inch below the skin in the calf. The needle can be clearly seen on x-ray and "seems" as if it could be easily localized and removed in the ER. However, after 30 minutes of probing around, the only result is a screaming child, a bloody leg, and a sweaty, embarrassed physician with no needle. Therefore, buried foreign objects should be removed in the operating room. There, you can use adequate anesthesia, good hemostasis, appropriate lighting, and necessary tools (curved hemostats and mini–x-ray units) so that the entire process takes 10 minutes and becomes technically simple. Furthermore, buried objects in the hand are often only a few millimeters away from blood vessels and nerves, and injudicious probing is more likely to produce injury than to find the target object.

Identification of Objects

Metal objects are the easiest to identify because they show up on x-ray. Other common foreign objects include wood, gravel, plastic, and glass. The best way to characterize the size and location of these materials is with a computed tomography scan.

Wood is notoriously troublesome. Large wood splinters often break apart when the patient attempts to remove them. Often left behind are residual wood fragments that may even be bigger than the piece the patient initially removed. Many times there is no substitute for operative exploration of the site. Do not be fooled into performing such an exploration in a nonoperative setting.

Large Objects

You may see patients with large, dramatic foreign-object injuries, such a steak knife stuck all the way through the forearm. In these cases, it is often appropriate to take the patient to the operating room immediately and remove the offending object. Large items (e.g., knives, hunting arrows, machine parts) can often tamponade blood vessels that have been severed, and removal may produce dramatic hemorrhage. Furthermore, large-object penetration frequently produces injuries that require nerve, vessel, or tendon repair. This care is often best administered immediately in an operating room environment.

GUNSHOT WOUNDS

Understanding gunshot wounds depends partially on a knowledge of ballistics.

Velocity

The energy represented by a projectile is proportional to its mass and the *square* of its velocity. A bigger projectile (larger mass) will do more damage, but increasing the projectile's speed can be devastating, because doubling the speed increases the representative energy by a factor of 4. Therefore, guns that have higher muzzle velocities produce dramatic injuries. Hunting rifles as well as military assault weapons commonly produce muzzle velocities in the range of 3000 feet per second, and a single shot from such a weapon can transfer enough energy to result in loss of a limb.

Bullet Design

As the projectile (bullet) travels through tissue, a shock wave is produced that causes secondary damage to adjacent tissue. The size and nature of the shock wave depend on the speed (energy) of the bullet as well as the bullet's motion characteristics. For example, some bullets are designed to crumple on impact, which causes their shape to "mushroom," and the wound features assume a tearing, irregular appearance (as opposed to a clean hole being drilled through the extremity). Some bullets are designed to "tumble" end over end as they travel through tissue, which also causes considerable collateral damage. In the open-fracture classification of Gustillo and Anderson, fracture due to a high-velocity gunshot wound qualifies as a type III injury (see Chapter 1).

Exit Wound

Remember that the entry wound of a bullet is often small and unimpressive, regardless of muzzle velocity

198 The Emergency Room

and bullet design. The exit wound, however, may be impressive, if not spectacularly large, in cases of high-speed guns or destructive bullet types. Also, be aware that bone and other structures can alter the bullet's path, so that the exit wound may not be in a straight line with the entry wound.

Obtain x-rays of all tissues near the bullet pathway. In some situations, there may be no exit wound and the bullet (or fragments of it) may be easily localized on x-ray. Carefully document the neurovascular status of the involved limb, because even if an artery is not transected by the projectile, shock-wave damage to a vessel's intima can produce thrombosis.

Bullet Fragments

Even though many bullet fragments may populate the soft tissues, there is usually little indication to remove a bullet or its fragments unless the pieces are causing neurovascular compromise or reside in a synovial space (or the spinal canal). In patients in whom the bullet produces no specific nerve, vessel, or tendon damage, care may be limited to simply débriding the entry and exit wounds and proceeding with routine antibiotic and tetanus prophylaxis. Shotgun shells, in particular, leave dozens of pellets in the soft tissues; attempting to remove them is rarely indicated and exposes the patient to a higher risk of inadvertently damaging normal structures.

Shotgun Injuries

Shotgun injuries deserve additional special mention for two reasons:

1. Close-range shotgun blasts represent huge energy transfers and can literally blow off a limb.
2. The material, or "wadding," that is used to pack shotgun shells is often refuse such as animal cartilage, and a shotgun blast can introduce this material deeply into the wound. This material should be considered highly contaminated because it has the potential to produce dramatic infection.

POWER-TOOL WOUNDS

Like gunshot wounds, power-tool injuries represent high-energy trauma. Ascertaining exactly how the accident happened and what type of machinery was involved can be helpful. Identification of the type of saw blade and material being cut before the accident, for example, may tell you about the type of foreign material likely to be embedded in the wound and whether the injury margins will be clean or ragged. Punch presses, table saws, and power drills commonly produce this type of injury.

High-pressure injection injuries merit special mention. This injury is related to high-pressure devices such as paint guns, in which a large amount of paint or solvent can be injected under high pressure in an instant. Wounds from this type of tool typically appear as tiny puncture marks. However, even if the puncture mark is in the fingertip, paint may be injected as high as the elbow because of the high pressures involved. These are devastating injuries because the material injected is usually quite locally toxic and difficult to remove. Wide-open débridement of the entire extremity may be required, and the likelihood of amputation is significant.

WOUNDS OF THE HAND

Tendon Lacerations

Extensor tendons can sometimes be easily repaired in the ER, especially if both ends of the involved tendon can be directly visualized. Flexor tendon repair, however, is more difficult because of the anatomy of the pulley system (zone 2) and the close proximity of neurovascular structures to the tendons. *Flexor tendon repair is reserved for the operating room environment.*

Open Dislocations

Occasionally, a dislocated finger undergoes enough deformity at the time of injury that the skin and subcutaneous tissues tear apart, yielding an open dislocation.

Because the dislocation is often reduced immediately (sometimes by the patient), this injury may manifest only as a transverse skin laceration in the finger, typically at the proximal interphalangeal joint flexion crease. You can detect such a laceration by testing the joint for stability and pursuing the patient's injury history.

Open lacerations represent open-joint injuries, and many authors believe that operative débridement significantly reduces the likelihood of infection. This is partly due to the fact that dirt or other foreign material can be easily sucked into the wound or joint during the reduction process.

Fingertip Amputations

Amputations of the fingertip are very common injuries, and most physicians hate taking care of them. The patient (and his or her family) is often quite upset because of the dramatic appearance of the fingertip. Common mechanisms of injury are car doors, window edges, folding chairs, and door jambs. Toddlers are particularly prone to putting their fingers where they do not belong.

The following are guidelines for managing a patient with a fingertip amputation:

1. Identify what is damaged. Nailbed lacerations should be repaired, which requires removal of the nail plate to view the laceration.
2. Repair the nail laceration. A digital block using local anesthetic is perfect for this procedure. The nail plate is quite securely attached distally and can be easily removed by using a small curved hemostat to bluntly spread underneath it. Often the proximal part of the nail plate will have dislocated out of the nail fold because the proximal area of the nailbed (germinal matrix) holds the nail plate less securely than the distal nailbed (sterile matrix). Repair of the nailbed is important because this tissue acts as a guide for nail-plate formation and growth. Nailbed lacerations should be repaired with tiny sutures (6-0 or 7-0 size), and using an absorbable suture is helpful so that suture removal will not be necessary.

3. Prop open, or "stent open," the proximal nail fold (eponychial fold). If this fold is not kept open for the first week or so after injury, it can scar down to the proximal nailbed and prevent a new nail from growing distally. Usually, a piece of adaptic gauze (or even the removed nail plate, if it is clean) can be used to stent open the nail fold.

4. In more severe injuries, the distal phalanx will be broken. No specific intervention is necessary if the tuft is crushed, because the tuft will reliably reconstitute over several months. However, often pinning is required if the distal phalangeal shaft is broken and if the fingertip is grossly unstable or deformed. The pinning process and nailbed repair are then best accomplished in the operating room.

5. The most severe fingertip injuries result in actual amputation of the tip. The pattern of amputation may be perfectly transverse, or it may be oblique such that there is more tissue left on either the dorsal or the volar side of the stump. In cases in which there is adequate tissue (either volarly or laterally), a variety of clever advancement flaps have been described to provide immediate coverage of the stump. Other coverage options include skin grafts and cross-finger flaps. Although certain types of finger wounds merit these procedures, a large body of literature supports the "open-wound" method of managing most distal tip amputations. The open-wound protocol involves covering the stump with a piece of nonadherent gauze and performing daily dressing changes. This method avoids the complications associated with flap and grafting procedures and reliably produces a cosmetically and functionally excellent result by comparison.

6. Inform all patients with crushed or amputated fingertips that they may experience hypersensitivity to touch and cold intolerance of the affected digit for up to 2 years after the injury date.

For the more severe injuries, early involvement of a hand therapist may be helpful to promote toughening of the stump, joint motion, and sensory desensitization.

9
CHAPTER

Infections

The orthopaedic surgeon is frequently the main consultant asked to evaluate and manage infections that occur in the extremities or initially derive from open wounds. This chapter reviews several of the classic infection scenarios. Although some of these situations represent merely a nuisance to the patient and doctor, a few of these processes can quickly become limb- or life-threatening. The clinical presentation usually begins in the emergency room (ER). Postoperative wound infections and toxic shock syndrome are covered in Chapter 13, and bite-wound infections are discussed in Chapter 8.

GAS GANGRENE

Gas gangrene has also been termed *clostridial myonecrosis* because this process is most commonly due to bacteria of the clostridial species. The most common specific organism is *Clostridium perfringens*. The virulence of the infection and resultant muscle necrosis are related to the production of lethal exotoxins. Once these exotoxins are disseminated, rapid muscle and soft-tissue liquefaction occurs and is associated with high mortality. Therefore, prevention and early detection are crucial.

Clostridia bacteria are gram-positive, anaerobic, spore-forming bacilli. They thrive in environments with low oxygen tension and necrotic tissue. Although *C. perfringens* is commonly found in fecal matter, it can be found almost everywhere, including the skin and hospital corridors. Its ability to cause infection is less related to intrinsic virulence and more dependent on ideal conditions in host tissue that allow bacteria growth and toxin production. Dirty wounds that are sutured tightly (or open fractures that are sealed with tight casts) represent contaminated tissues that can become ischemic (or poorly oxygenated), and it is this environment that frequently sets the stage for clostridial infection. Deep wounds into muscular areas (buttock, thigh, shoulder) are classic locations.

Once clostridial replication starts, lethal histotoxins are produced that cause cell wall destruction with subsequent local tissue death. This widens the zone of low oxygen tension and necrosis, allowing greater clostridial growth and advancing colonization.

Clinical Presentation

The particular character of the wound and host characterize the situation in which clostridial myonecrosis can develop. Preconditions for developing gas gangrene are (1) dirty wounds that are sealed, (2) wounds that deeply penetrate muscular areas, and (3) compromised hosts (i.e., diabetics, immunosuppressed patients).

The key to clinical diagnosis is severe pain and local swelling in the face of dramatic tissue destruction. Gas formation may not be particularly dramatic or even present in some cases. Any drainage fluid should be gram-stained, looking in particular for gram-positive bacilli.

The clinical scenario is characterized by rapid deterioration. The incubation period for clostridia is only 12 to 24 hours after injury, and patients usually complain first of severe pain. Tachycardia without significant fever is also an early finding, and the wound typically is swollen and draining serous, hemorrhagic fluid. The process spreads quickly, and the affected limb may soon look tense and white or bronze and exude a musty odor.

X-rays of the limb may show the classic gas production, which appears as numerous small bubbles within muscular zones. The actual extent of necrotic muscle is often much greater than might appear on physical exam, and patients can quickly become comatose and die.

Diagnostic Considerations

The gas due to clostridial myonecrosis tends to be bubbly and located within muscle planes. A variety of infections can produce gas, however, including anaerobic cellulitis and streptococcal infections. Therefore, the presence of gas alone is not enough to make a specific diagnosis, although gas formation due to infection is generally a good clue that a severe, possibly limb- or life-threatening infection should be considered.

Another issue is that the presence of gas (e.g., air) in a soft-tissue plane does not necessarily mean that infection is present. For example, any penetrating wound has the potential to introduce a small amount of air into the deep tissues, and this will occasionally be obvious on x-ray. Dog bites frequently result in pockets of air within the wound, because these wounds are commonly produced through a tearing and ripping mechanism. Sometimes the ER staff or the radiologist will call you specifically to point out that x-rays of your next patient (whom you have not yet seen) have shown gas in the soft tissues. Do not to jump to conclusions. Most of the air in soft-tissue planes seen on films of acute wounds is due to air introduction at the time of wounding. Although your respect for gas gangrene can never be too great, gas formation due to infection requires that an established infection be present at least for a short period.

Treatment

Treatment of gas gangrene consists of the following methods:

1. **Complete débridement of dead tissue:** This is the most critical element of treatment. Multiple large incisions may be necessary to perform the radical removal of infected muscle. Unless the diagnosis is made relatively early, amputation of the affected limb may be necessary to save the patient's life.

2. **Antibiotics:** Penicillin is the antibiotic of choice. It is often administered as 3 million U IV q3h. Other organisms not uncommonly superinfect the areas of dead tissue, and a second antibiotic, such as an aminoglycoside, is often added to the penicillin regimen.
3. **Fluid resuscitation:** Fluid loss due to myonecrosis and toxin circulation requires aggressive support, including the monitoring of central venous pressure and urinary output.
4. **Oxygen administration:** Hyperbaric oxygen treatments may also be helpful, because clostridia organisms do poorly if the tissue oxygen tension is high. Unfortunately, many hospitals do not have hyperbaric oxygen chambers, and transferring the patient to such a location must be weighed against time lost in the transfer process.

Remember that gas gangrene can quickly become limb and life threatening. Early recognition and treatment with surgical débridement and massive fluid and antibiotic support are key to preventing morbidity and mortality.

NECROTIZING FASCIITIS

Necrotizing fasciitis is another highly destructive infectious process that can be fatal. It can be caused by a variety of bacteria, although hemolytic group A streptococcus is the most common offender. Immunocompromised patients as well as IV drug abusers and alcoholics seem to be at particular risk.

The clinical presentation typically starts as a cellulitis that progresses rapidly and does not respond well to the usual support of antibiotics and elevation. Eventually skin blistering occurs and then necrosis of the skin and subcutaneous tissues follows. Muscle tissue is typically not involved in necrotizing fasciitis (in contradistinction to gas gangrene).

Treatment mandates radical surgical débridement of involved tissue planes. Extensive longitudinal incisions are often necessary, and necrotic skin, fat, and thrombosed vessels must be removed. Giant open wounds are the usual result of adequate surgical management, and these may be covered with skin grafts once the infection is cleared.

TETANUS

Knowledge about tetanus is important because every patient you see with a laceration should have their tetanus immunization status checked. Although tetanus is a potentially fatal disease, it is easy to prevent. This infection is caused by another species of *Clostridium*, specifically *C. tetani*. Even though this organism is a strict anaerobe (gram-positive bacillus), it can colonize superficial wounds. The clinical manifestations of tetanus are caused by toxins produced during an established infection.

Tetanus spores are found primarily in fecal matter and soil. They are very resistant organisms, and several hours of boiling are required to kill them (or 10 minutes in the autoclave). Any type of wound can be susceptible to tetanus infection, although ischemia and coexisting infection increase the odds.

Clinical Presentation

The clinical presentation of tetanus relates to the production and dissemination of neurotoxins that are carried through the peripheral nerves to the central nervous system. Voluntary muscle groups seem to be affected the most, and toxin-bound muscle results in severe spasm.

The incubation period has been reported to be approximately 1 week, and an early sign of toxin production may be muscle spasm near the site of injury. Subsequently, pharyngeal and facial muscles are classically involved, the former accounting for tetanus's nickname of "lockjaw." The mortality rate for those patients exhibiting the full blown clinical disease is greater than 50 percent, and death usually results from respiratory arrest due to paralysis of the laryngeal and respiratory muscles.

Treatment and Prevention

Treatment involves massive doses of penicillin and tetanus immune globulin, débridement of the inciting wound, and supportive care, particularly of the respiratory system.

Tetanus can be reliably prevented by appropriate immunization. Although the ER staff generally ask patients with a wound about their last tetanus booster, do not assume that this has been done. Make a point of asking the patient yourself. In the United States, most children have been vaccinated through their school program. Ask anyway. For adults, the key question is when they had their last tetanus booster shot. If the patient cannot remember, assume that they never had one.

The specific algorithm that describes when and how much immunization should be administered depends on the type of wound and when the patient was last immunized. The details of an accepted protocol are noted in Table 9–1. Although you may not actually give any of these injections yourself, you should understand the protocol and appreciate the importance of making sure that patients are immunized properly.

SEPTIC ARTHRITIS

Infection within a joint space must be treated emergently because irreversible destruction of articular cartilage occurs quickly. Joints may be infected by direct traumatic penetration or hematogenous transmission of bacteria can seed the intra-articular space.

Clinical Presentation

The patient's history may be particularly relevant because underlying medical conditions that compromise the host response to infection often play a role in the infection's genesis. Furthermore, medication usage should be elicited to document whether corticosteroids or other immunosuppression drugs may be at work.

Physical findings are marked swelling and a tense effusion of the affected joint. Warmth and skin changes, even frank cellulitis, may be present as well. Severe

Table 9–1. TETANUS IMMUNIZATION: GENERAL GUIDELINES

Clinical Situation	Immunization Recommendation
PREVIOUSLY IMMUNIZED PATIENT: ACTIVELY IMMUNIZED WITHIN PAST 10 YEARS	
Patient has received a booster within past 5 years	Nothing new required
Patient has NOT received a booster within the past 5 years	Administer 0.5 mL of adsorbed tetanus toxoid as a booster
PREVIOUSLY IMMUNIZED PATIENT: ACTIVELY IMMUNIZED MORE THAN 10 YEARS PRIOR	
For routine wounds	Administer 0.5 mL of adsorbed tetanus toxoid as a booster
For severe, neglected, or old (more than 24 hours) tetanus-prone wounds	1. Administer 0.5 mL of adsorbed tetanus toxoid 2. Also administer 250 units of tetanus immune globulin (human) 3. Consider administration of oxytetracycline or penicillin

FOR PATIENTS NOT PREVIOUSLY IMMUNIZED

For clean, minor wounds in which tetanus is unlikely	Administer 0.5 mL of adsorbed tetanus toxoid
All other wounds	1. Administer 0.5 mL of adsorbed tetanus toxoid
	2. Administer 250 units of tetanus immune globulin (human); give 500 units if the wound is severe, neglected, or more than 24 hours old
	3. Consider administration of oxytetracycline or penicillin

Note: a) Some experts recommend 6 years instead of 10 as the acceptable time limit for active immunization, especially with neglected or particularly tetanus-prone wounds.
b) When administering tetanus toxoid as well as tetanus immune globulin, use different syringes, needles, and injection locations.
c) Appropriate tetanus prophylaxis includes standard wound care regardless of the patient's immunization status. This means cleaning the wound, removing dead tissue and foreign bodies, and surgical care if indicated.

pain will likely be the patient's main complaint, and the affected joint will tend to be held in a position that produces the least intracapsular pressure. This position is usually one of partial flexion for the elbow, knee, and ankle. Flexion with external rotation is often the most comfortable position for the hip. Spectacular tenderness can typically be elicited by passive motion on physical exam. In fact, just a small amount of motion is usually quite painful if the joint is infected. Another helpful physical finding will be tenderness around the entire circumference of the joint. For example, an infected knee will be tender to palpation and tensely swollen when examined both medially and laterally.

The patient's vital signs, especially the presence of fever, and routine laboratory studies should be checked. Relevant studies include a white blood cell count, sedimentation rate, and blood cultures. Plain x-rays should be obtained, both to identify whether there are any foreign bodies in the joint (e.g., arthroplasty components) and to assess whether or not there is any evidence of bone destruction consistent with osteomyelitis. If the index of suspicion is high for infection, the simplest and most definitive diagnostic tool is aspiration of the joint. Avoid aspirating a joint through infected skin, so that you do not introduce bacteria and make matters worse. If gross pus is retrieved or if the Gram stain is positive, intervention should be started as soon as possible.

Treatment

Treatment of the septic joint usually requires the following procedures:

1. **Operative drainage:** In some situations, repeated aspiration also has been thought to be effective. However, most patients who are healthy enough to tolerate an anesthetic usually end up in the operating room. Some joints, such as the knee and shoulder, are particularly amenable to arthroscopic irrigation and débridement, and this may frequently be the method by which surgical drainage is accomplished.
2. **Antibiotics:** IV antibiotics are also part of the treatment routine. If no good culture specimen has been

obtained before operative intervention and if operative intervention will occur within 1 or 2 hours of presentation, it may make sense to hold off on starting antibiotics until a good sample of infected fluid or tissue is obtained. That way, it may be easier to grow the offending organism in culture and identify the bacterial organism. Antibiotics would then be administered immediately after the sample is obtained. If, however, the patient cannot be treated with drainage immediately, antibiotics should be started even if a sample of joint fluid cannot be obtained so that therapy is instituted promptly.

Special Populations at Risk

Certain patient populations are at particular risk for specific infections. Pediatric patients represent one such population. Children in general are at risk for hematogenous spread of infection to the joint space because of the rich metaphyseal blood supply that characterizes the growing skeleton. The most common organism overall is *Staphylococcus aureus.* Infection in neonates is frequently due to group B streptococcus; in the 6- to 48-month-old age group, *Haemophilus influenzae* is often the offending bacteria.

Note that a septic joint in a child, particularly in an infant, can be extremely difficult to diagnose. The physical exam may be unimpressive except for the presence of a limp or refusal to bear weight on the limb. In an infant, nothing more than loss of appetite and "irritability" may be present. The correct diagnosis is crucial because a septic hip often requires operative drainage to avoid long-term developmental abnormalities. Be aware of infection as a possible diagnosis in any baby who presents with irritability and evidence of extremity discomfort or reluctance to move normally. In some situations, an immediate ultrasound exam of the hip or even direct needle aspiration of the hip joint may be necessary to thoroughly rule out the possibility of a septic joint.

Neisseria gonorrhoeae is the most common bacterial organism to produce septic arthritis in young adults, and another clue to this process is the presence of skin papules. Other populations of patients at particular risk include those with diabetes, rheumatoid arthritis, or drug abuse problems, those on dialysis, and anyone else who is immunocompromised.

SEPTIC FLEXOR TENOSYNOVITIS

Infection within the digital flexor tendon sheath constitutes an emergency, similar to that of an infected joint. The Zone II flexion tendon pathway, which constitutes the area in the finger where the sublimus and profundus flexor tendons share occupancy within the pulley system, does not tolerate additional volume (Fig. 9–1). The flexor tendons fit perfectly in this space, and normal flexor function relies on gliding between the tendons and the pulley walls. Infection in this space quickly exceeds the critical volume limits of the space and also produces an inflammatory response that can permanently destroy the tendon's ability to glide. Aside from actually producing liquefaction of the tendons themselves, even mild or short-lived infections can stimulate a scar response that can, for all practical purposes, cause the flexor tendons to become glued together or irrevocably stuck to the tendon sheath walls.

Flexor tendon infections are usually caused by a puncture wound somewhere along the digital flexor's pathway, often in the finger or possibly in the distal palm. Again, similar to the felon, the inciting wound may be small enough that it heals by the time the patient presents for treatment, and no obvious portal of entry can be found.

Clinical Presentation

Septic flexor tenosynovitis is manifested clinically by several classic findings, referred to as the "four cardinal signs of Kanavel":

1. Uniform swelling of the involved digit
2. Partially flexed posture of the affected digit
3. Severe tenderness along the pathway of the tendon within the tendon sheath
4. Severe pain along the tendon sheath pathway caused by passive extension of the finger

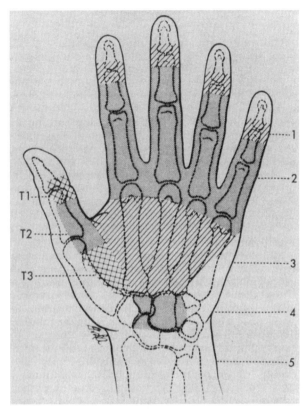

Figure 9–1. Diagram illustrating the various flexor tendon zones, drawn according to the recommendations of the Flexor Tendon Committee of the International Federation of Societies for Surgery of the Hand (IFSSH).

These signs all relate to the presence of pus within the confined space of the tendon sheath. All four signs do not need to be present to make the diagnosis of septic flexor tenosynovitis, although usually several of the signs are present at a minimum. Probably the most reliable sign is tenderness along the entire tendon pathway, not just in one location in the digit.

Treatment

The most common offending organisms are skin flora, specifically *S. aureus*. If infection is suspected within the flexor tendon sheath, aggressive management must be undertaken. If the patient presents within the first 24 to 48 hours and has only mild findings, sometimes IV antibiotics will be adequate. The patient should, however, be admitted and have the hand immobilized and elevated. Careful scrutiny of the clinical course is required to make sure that the process is improving.

If improvement does not occur obviously and quickly or if the patient presents with advanced findings or more than 48 hours of symptoms, surgical drainage is usually best. It is critical not to allow the infection to get out of control and destroy the delicate balance within the tendon sheath system.

Surgical drainage may require a major, volar, zigzag-type incision involving the entire digit and palm if advanced infection is present. It is sometimes possible to effect satisfactory surgical drainage by making a proximal (distal palmar crease) and distal (distal interphalangeal flexion crease) incision and then irrigating the tendon system through these two incisions. The use of a small-diameter red-rubber catheter can facilitate finger irrigation through these two incisions. It is important to ensure that adequate volume can be exchanged through the finger so that satisfactory cleaning is accomplished. If there is any doubt or difficulty with a limited approach, a wider incision should be used. Be aware that any attempt at draining a septic flexor tenosynovitis should be undertaken in an operating room environment.

After surgical drainage, a drain is usually left in place to prevent the reaccumulation of additional pus. Patients with this injury frequently have very high hand therapy requirements, because early motion is key to their recovery and because postoperative pain often reduces their enthusiasm to move the finger.

PARONYCHIA

A paronychia is an infection of the tissues surrounding the nail fold. It is relatively common, and often the ER staff will treat it without consulting the orthopaedic surgery service. However, you will be asked to address this problem from time to time, and you should know how to deal with it.

For a paronychia to start, bacteria typically enter through an opening underneath the nail fold. Common mechanisms include nail biting, aggressive manicures, and hangnail-related lacerations. Patients notice redness and swelling of the nail fold and, often within 1 or 2 days, develop enough pain that the problem cannot be ignored. Skin organisms are the usual offenders, with *S. aureus* being the most common.

Treatment

Treatment depends on drainage. A metacarpal block with 1 percent lidocaine (Xylocaine) will provide satisfactory anesthesia. If the abscess is localized to one area of the nail fold, simply spreading the fold open with a small hemostat allows pus to drain out. Placement of a small piece of gauze under the fold will help to keep the area open to facilitate further drainage. The patient can then pursue a course of warm soaks at home to ensure resolution. Oral antibiotics are also advisable for a week or so.

If the paronychia has been present for some time, it may extend to both sides of the nail fold or actually penetrate beneath the nail plate and elevate it off the nailbed. In these cases, removal of the nail plate is required to adequately decompress the infected area. On occasion an incision is necessary to drain deeper abscess formation, but be careful about indiscriminately incising the nailbed itself because this can lead to deformity of future nail-plate growth.

FELON

A felon is an infection involving the pulp space of a finger. The pulp space has relatively limited volume capacity, bordered proximally by the distal interphalangeal flexion crease. The skin and subcutaneous tissues are firmly attached distally and peripherally and contribute to the "closed-space" character of the pulp.

Felons are usually caused by a puncture wound or deep laceration. Sometimes the original wound heals quickly, and by the time the patient presents with a pulp-space infection, there appears to be no inciting wound.

Clinical presentation is characterized by swelling and redness of the finger pad. The patient is usually experiencing intense pain. The pain derives from increasing pressure (pus) accumulating in a closed space, and often the finger pad is tense enough to feel rock hard.

The most common organisms responsible for this condition are skin flora.

Treatment

Treatment of a felon relies on (1) drainage of the abscess and (2) keeping the wound open with a wick so that continued drainage is possible. Initial antibiotic coverage should cover skin organisms, but obtain cultures of the drainage so that exact identification of the inciting bug can be confirmed.

Drainage involves making an incision in the fingertip. There are a wide variety of recommendations as to the best spot for making the cut. Clearly, you should not make an incision that destabilizes the finger pad or is placed in such a way that the scar itself will be chronically tender. One acceptable location is on the volar finger pad, with the incision being longitudinal and no more proximally extended than the flexion crease. The other location, which may be even better, is a laterally located incision, just volar to the nail cuticle. Do not cross over to the midaxial line of the digit if you use the lateral incision, and do not place the lateral incision too volar so that it is truly in the midlateral line of the finger. Both these errors tend to destabilize the finger pad (and possibly devascularize it) by violating the vertical septa within the finger pad's internal structure.

Whichever incision location you pick, make sure it is directly over (or at least very close to) the part of the finger that is most swollen and most likely to contain the pus. Occasionally, two incisions may be necessary, one on each side of the digit. Be very careful not to destabilize the finger pad. Sometimes it will be necessary to use a small hemostat and spread within the pulp space to facilitate drainage. Do this carefully.

WHITLOW

Whitlow is a herpes simplex viral infection of the fingertip. It commonly presents in both children and adults. The classic history relates to the patient's occupation as either a dental hygienist or a respiratory care therapist. You need to know about this process because it often presents with a dramatic clinical picture, which, ironically, requires no invasive management. The infection is self-limited and resolves without any intervention within 2 to 4 weeks.

Clinical Presentation

Patients demonstrate white, fluid-filled blisters that eventually fuse together and then disappear. Swelling and redness of the fingertip can be dramatic, and patients usually present to the ER because of terrific pain in the finger.

Unfortunately, some patients with whitlow do not present when their blisters are present, and the severe erythema and crusty, draining skin mimic the appearance of a bacterial infection. Many patients undergo incision in an effort to drain a presumed abscess. Invasion of the finger, however, makes the process worse and has no effect on the viral course. It merely opens an already compromised zone of skin to allow skin bacteria a better portal of entry. Patients with whitlow who undergo incision often become superinfected with *S. aureus*, thereby greatly increasing the complexity of management.

The viral process tends to be very superficial, and usually only the skin and underlying subcutaneous tissues are involved. Health-care workers with a reddened, tender, blistering finger should be highly suspected of having this viral infection. Even if no blisters are present, ask the patient about his or her occupation to ascertain whether he or she is at risk for exposure to oral secretions.

Treatment

If you do see a patient when blisters are present, the fluid within contains viral material, so wear gloves and wash your hands. Some authors advocate draining the blisters to improve pain, but this does not shorten the disease course.

Treatment of whitlow is supportive. Sometimes narcotic pain medication is necessary for a few days. Oral antibiotics probably do not make any difference, but if you suspect that a bacterial component is also present, antibiotics probably will not hurt. Antiviral agents, such as acyclovir, may be helpful in shortening the time to resolution, but they must be started within the first few days of onset to make a difference.

Operative care is indicated only if it is clear that a bacterial abscess is present. It can be very difficult to resist incising the finger because the patient can present in considerable distress. The digit is red, swollen, very tender, and looks terrible, with crusting, blistering skin lesions at the peak of the process. Keep in mind that incising the virally infected finger will not help and will only increase the potential for deeper infection or introduce bacteria. Consider swabbing the finger and sending the culture to the viral laboratory, which may confirm the diagnosis.

Patient education may help if the viral infection recurs.

LYME DISEASE

Lyme disease is the most common insect-carried illness in the United States and is due to a gram-negative spirochete called *Borrelia burgdorferi*, which is carried by the deer tick, *Ixodes dammini*. You may occasionally be called to evaluate rashes and cellulitic processes in the extremities, and this is one diagnosis you should keep in mind. Lyme disease is common in parts of the country that have a large deer or rodent population (northeast, middle Atlantic, north central, and Pacific coastal areas). Be aware that the process may not appear for up to a month after a tick bite, so patients who have traveled through high-risk geographical areas may

Table 9–2. THE STAGES OF LYME DISEASE

Stage I—early localized infection; occurs within 3 to 30 days after a tick bite and manifests as an expanding erythematous ring with a centrally clear zone (called *erythema chronicum migrans*). Also present will be moderate swelling in one or more joints.

Stage II—early disseminated infection; results in neurologic manifestations (including facial nerve paralysis) and cardiac problems. Also evident may be migratory joint pain without dramatic swelling.

Stage III—persistent infection; occurs within 6 mo and involves progression to arthritic complications, most commonly in large joints such as the knee. Episodes of pain and dramatic effusions initially last a few days, but after several years, may be months in duration. Of untreated patients, about 20% develop chronic Lyme arthritis, which denotes continuous joint involvement for more than 1 year.

have been exposed even though their home location does not suggest high risk.

The most common laboratory test used to identify the process (enzyme-linked immunosorbent assay) is highly sensitive and specific, but only late in the disease course. Early in the disease, the patient's erythrocyte sedimentation rate will be high. Clinical findings such as the characteristic rash may be the best initial clue.

Lyme disease has three stages, listed in Table 9–2. Treatment of stages I and II disease depends on antibiotics. Oral administration of amoxicillin for 1 month may be adequate if the disease is not too severely advanced. Lyme arthritis may require intravenous antibiotics and possibly intra-articular corticosteroid administration and synovectomy in severe cases.

GONOCOCCAL INFECTIONS

Strange as it may seem, orthopaedic surgeons do become involved in diagnosing sexually transmitted disease. This is because the most common cause of septic arthritis in young adults is *N. gonorrhoeae* infection. Women are affected four times more frequently than men. Initial presentation includes a low-grade fever, chills, and the sudden onset of migratory arthralgias. The process can present primarily as a bacteremia, in which fever and chills are accompanied by dermatitis (or skin papules) and tenosynovitis. Alternatively, patients may be affected by the suppurative form of gonorrhea, in which joint involvement is the major manifestation.

You must consider gonococcal infection in any young adult with a suspected septic joint. Unfortunately, diagnosis can be difficult because only 50 percent of infected joints yield a positive culture, and blood cultures are often negative as well. Cultures of the genitourinary tract provide the highest yield. Although it is appropriate to ask about a vaginal or urethral discharge or dysuria, many patients may be without these symptoms.

Treatment

Treatment of gonorrhea consists of appropriate antibiotic therapy. Because so many *N. gonorrhoeae* strains are penicillin resistant, a β-lactamase–resistant cephalosporin (e.g., ceftriaxone) is often administered. The presence of joint purulence requires hospital admission, although open surgical drainage is rarely required except for the hip. *Complete management includes issues of patient education and treatment of the patient's sexual contacts.*

CELLULITIS

Cellulitis refers to infection of the skin and subcutaneous tissues, most frequently caused by *Staphylococcus* or *Streptococcus* species. The orthopaedic surgery service is often consulted for this problem, either when the patient first presents to the ER or after initial treatment has failed.

Clinical Assessment

The hallmarks of the physical exam are local redness, swelling, and tenderness over the reddened areas. Lymphangitis, as demonstrated by a proximally spreading red streak, may also be present. Host factors play a role in the speed and severity of infection; in already compromised patients, cellulitis can produce significant tissue loss and sepsis.

The most common scenario is one in which a previously healthy person sustains a cut or insect bite and then later notices progressive swelling and redness of the skin. In many cases, the ER staff may send the patient home with a course of oral antibiotics and skincare education, and in many of these cases, the process ends. However, for those who do not respond to this initial treatment plan, you will be called. Any significant amount of skin redness or advancing lymphangitis usually requires hospital admission. (Attempts to avoid admission in these circumstances just prolong the total treatment time, because hospitalization generally becomes an obvious requirement the next day when the cellulitis has worsened.)

Treatment

There are three key elements in treating advanced cellulitis.

1. **Intravenous antibiotic therapy:** Make sure a reasonable antibiotic is chosen. Nafcillin is a favorite of the medical service, but note that it can be caustic to local tissues if it extravasates. A first-generation cephalosporin, such as cefazolin (Kefzol), also usually works well; it is inexpensive and well tolerated and provides nice coverage of common skin organisms.
2. **Immobilization of the affected part:** You may be consulted to assess a cellulitis case that is slow to respond and find the patient in the hospital room eating, holding the phone, and writing letters with the cellulitic hand. Such activity just adds irritation to an already inflamed part. You should immobilize the affected part, preferably with a padded bandage supported by a plaster or Velcro splint.

3. **Elevation of the infected area:** This tends to help reduce pain and swelling. Sometimes the best way to elevate the forearm or hand is to support the arm with a long piece of stockinet gauze tied to an IV pole. In whatever way elevation is accomplished, encourage constant compliance, especially while the patient is sleeping.

If there seems to be any potential pocket of purulent material, this should be drained. However, usually no obvious pus is available for drainage or culture. Sometimes the use of a heating pad is helpful to increase blood flow to the affected part and to localize a small abscessed area or loosen wound eschars.

Cellulitis usually responds to intravenous antibiotics, immobilization, and elevation within several days. If a lymphangitic streak is present, its length and direction of progression can be used as a general barometer of how the cellulitis is responding. Even if the streak rapidly diminishes, do not send the patient home until all the original erythema is gone. Patients should generally be discharged with a 10-day course of oral antibiotics.

In situations in which the cellulitis does not seem to be improving despite standard aggressive care, additional factors should be considered. Perhaps an abscess is present that hasn't been identified. Consider, too, the host factors. Diabetes, skin disorders, and immune compromise are conditions that may make treatment more difficult.

Olecranon Cellulitis

Skin overlying the olecranon is redundant, so that terminal elbow flexion is not limited by skin tension. However, in extension, this skin and underlying bursa are lax and create a potential space. If a cellulitis starts in this area, associated swelling often is manifested by fluid engorgement of the underlying olecranon bursa. Patients then present with a golf ball–sized mass on the posterior elbow, which is really just the fluid-filled olecranon bursa.

A common scenario is that minimal cellulitis is present. The patient presents with the singular complaint of having a large, round mass on the back of the elbow. It is often assumed that some dramatic course of action is required based on the lesion's size. However, take a careful history and inspect the patient's elbow carefully. You will be surprised to discover that absolutely no pain is present, full elbow range of motion exists, and the patient has had this lesion for about a month. This common scenario requires no invasive care. In fact, attempting to drain the bursa, however tempting it might be, merely exposes the patient to a small, but definite, risk of contaminating the space and converting a relatively asymptomatic fluid collection into a disaster. Drainage and corticosteroid injection are usually not helpful anyway because the fluid usually returns within 24 hours. Furthermore, if a small amount of cellulitis is present, you are ill advised to inject any area through this infected skin.

Following are key treatment points for managing the patient with olecranon bursitis:

1. Treatment depends on whether an infection is present. If the overlying skin is red and tender, management is the same as for any cellulitis: antibiotics, immobilization, and elevation. If the bursa itself is loaded with pus, operative drainage is required.
2. Treatment of aseptic olecranon bursitis should address the underlying cause. Usually, this is a combination of dry, cracked skin (which facilitates a mild cellulitis) and repeated, inadvertent trauma to the elbow (e.g., resting on an armrest, bumping into a wall, abrasive clothing). Carpenters, construction workers, firemen, and other people who work around rough materials or ladders are often affected by olecranon bursitis.
3. After the cellulitis component has been treated, the fluid collection can be most safely managed by two modalities: (1) eliminating any direct contact of the elbow with an irritating surface and (2) gentle, constant, external compression.
4. Educating the patient not to rest on the elbow and to wear an elbow pad at work can be very helpful. External compression can be provided by a loosely wrapped Ace bandage around the elbow. A month or so of such care often results in complete resolution of the bursal fluid accumulation without the risk associated with needle aspiration.

10
CHAPTER

Closed Soft-Tissue Trauma

GENERAL PROCEDURES

Some of the most common problems that orthopaedic surgeons manage include muscle, ligament, and tendon injuries. Although a large part of these injuries can be managed with supportive, symptomatic care, you will be frequently asked to assess these patients when they first present to the emergency room (ER). It is important to be familiar with basic management principles so that you can provide appropriate initial treatment and advice.

Initial Supportive Care for Soft-Tissue Injuries

The hallmark of treatment is the "RICE" protocol (*r*est, *i*ce, *c*ompression, and *e*levation).

Rest

Rest for the lower extremity usually can be accomplished by protected weight bearing with the use of crutches or a walker. It is advisable to make sure that the patient knows how to use such assist devices before being discharged from the ER. Often an ER nurse gives the patient a quick review. Be aware that some patients can fall while attempting to use crutches and sustain a worse injury than the one they had. "Rest" for the upper extremity may be accomplished with a sling or splint, depending on the location of the injury.

Ice

Ice is helpful for reduction of swelling and is most effective when applied within the first 48 hours. Direct contact of ice on the skin for any more than a few minutes should be avoided, because this can produce frostbite. Application of a cold compress, such as ice wrapped in a thick towel, is safer. Several periods of ice application per day are also more effective than a single prolonged session in the ER.

Compression

Compression is also helpful in the reduction of swelling and pain. It is typically achieved through application of a compression bandage. This can easily be constructed by wrapping several rolls of cast padding around the affected part and then covering this with an elastic Ace-type bandage. The bulkier you make the bandage, the better it functions for pain relief and protection. The outer Ace bandage adds a little extra compression and serves to hold the whole bandage together. It is probably a good idea not to use the little metal clips that come with many Ace bandages because small children can swallow or cut themselves on these clips. Adhesive tape is the best way to secure the dressing, but use strips of tape instead of wrapping tape around the extremity circumferentially. Many Ace bandages now come with Velcro strips that supplant the use of metal clips. Several longitudinal strips of tape are still helpful because they tend to prevent the bandage from unraveling or bunching up within the first few days. Be aware of the following key points when applying a compression bandage:

1. Start by wrapping from the most distal part of the extremity and then work your way proximally. If you start in the reverse direction (proximally first), it is possible for the dressing to partially unwind, bunch up, and exert a tourniquet effect on the limb. There-

fore, start distally, either at the fingertips or at the toes.
2. When wrapping, extend the bandage proximally until you go a good distance past the injured area. The injured zone should ideally be within the middle zone of your dressing. For example, for a calf injury, start by wrapping at the toes and go all the way to the knee. If you just wrap around the injured area, the uncovered area distal to the calf tends to become swollen as the bandage applies a venous tourniquet effect.
3. Avoid bunching up the bandage too much in any one area, and similar to padding application for a cast, overlap each revolution of the padding or Ace bandage by 50 percent. Careful technique in bandage application can make a big difference in how the patient feels and how the allied medical staff perceive your general competence.

Elevation

Elevation is the last component of RICE, and it can be just as important as the other elements in controlling pain and swelling. The ideal level of elevation should be even with the patient's heart. This level neither unduly increases arterial inflow to the limb nor impedes venous outflow. Patients often note immediately how uncomfortable their sprained ankle feels if they hold their foot in a dependent position. Emphasize strict elevation of the foot in the first few days after an injury.

Pain Management

Pain management after a muscle strain or ligament sprain may require narcotic medication. It is certainly reasonable to provide patients with a prescription for acetaminophen with codeine, for example, when they leave the ER. However, meticulous adherence to a rest, icing, and elevation protocol often greatly decreases the requirements for pain medication. In fact, narcotic use may make patients sleepy, nauseated, or constipated (or all three). Experienced orthopaedic consultants often stress using medication as a helpful adjunct in pain control, relying primarily on elevation and immobility as the main treatment. Watch how much different a patient with an ankle sprain feels when the foot is hanging in the dependent position as opposed to being placed up on four pillows.

MUSCLE INJURIES

Most muscle injuries occur from a traction force or a direct blow. If the traction exceeds the muscle's capacity for excursion, muscle fibers tear. Such damage is often referred to as a *strain*. These stretching-type injuries occur most frequently at the myotendinous junction and in muscles that cross more than one joint, such as the gastrocnemius. A blunt trauma can also produce structural disruption within the muscle. This is commonly termed a *contusion*.

Clinical Presentation

Because most muscles have rich blood supplies, muscle injuries are often associated with dramatic bleeding and subsequent swelling, discoloration, and pain. Intramuscular hematoma can occasionally become large enough to precipitate a compartment syndrome, even in a space such as the thigh. Therefore, note carefully how much swelling is present, and document the neurovascular status of the extremity carefully. If the muscle has been completely ruptured, loss of active motion will also be present. However, many injuries that produce little or no physical interruption of the muscle can produce enough pain that the patient may be unable to demonstrate active function when first examined. Direct palpation of the muscle is often helpful, because a complete disruption of the muscle belly will be manifested by a palpable defect in soft-tissue contour.

Treatment

Muscle strains may be treated according to the RICE protocol. Resting the involved part may be accomplished with application of a splint. However, because the injured part is usually in the lower extremity, use of protected weight bearing with crutches is adequate. Ice in the first 48 hours will help with reduction of swelling, as will a gently wrapped compression bandage. It may help to educate the patient that muscle strains can require a very long time to recover, sometimes beyond 3 months. Persistent tightness and aching in the muscle group can usually be resolved through supervised physical therapy, although the details of each individual case will dictate whether therapy is necessary. Surgical repair of a muscle injury is rarely indicated and may be relevant only in patients whose entire muscle belly has ruptured and retracted, leaving a large gap.

Tennis Leg

An example of a common muscle strain is "tennis leg," a tear of the medial head of the gastrocnemius from its origin behind the knee. Patients often describe running for a ball and then feeling a sharp, stabbing pain behind the knee, "as if I was shot in the leg." Clinical presentation demonstrates maintenance of active motion of the knee and ankle, although any movement that stretches the gastrocnemius produces significant pain. Symptomatic care and rest often allow the patient to return to normal activity within 6 to 8 weeks.

LIGAMENT INJURIES

Ligaments are stabilizing soft-tissue structures that connect one bone to another. A "sprain" refers to damage to the ligament, usually from a stretching-type mechanism. Sprains can be classified into the following types:

- Type I—mild injury with no gross disruption of the ligament attachment sites
- Type II—partial detachment of the ligament but with no significant instability of the bones involved
- Type III—complete disconnection of the ligament from one of its anchoring sites, which results in clinical instability of the joint

Clinical Presentation

The presentation of a sprain can be quite dramatic. Patients may have pain similar to that associated with fracture, and associated initial swelling can also be spectacular. Establish a mechanism of injury as carefully as possible, because this history may help identify some classic sprain-injury patterns. For example, inversion loading of the ankle is a typical mechanism for the common lateral ankle sprain.

On physical exam, palpate the affected joint carefully, because many times you will be able to precisely identify the affected ligament. This is where your knowledge of anatomy is crucial, because if you know the attachment sites for each specific ligament, you can quickly check them on physical exam and accurately assess the injury.

In differentiating a type III sprain from lesser injuries, stressing the joint to test for laxity may be helpful. This should be performed gently because it will be a painful maneuver. Sometimes injecting local anesthesia helps in facilitating the joint stressing part of the physical exam. Occasionally, it is helpful to obtain x-rays while the joint is being stressed ("stress views") because the films may more clearly document pathological joint laxity.

Radiographic Exam

Obtain plain x-rays to determine if a fracture is present. In fact, most patients are assumed to have a fracture based on the way their joint looks, and only when the films are negative is a sprain assumed to be the working diagnosis. Scrutinize the plain films carefully, because tiny bony avulsion fragments provide clues as to where the soft-tissue injury has occurred.

Initial Treatment

Initial treatment of the sprained joint follows the RICE protocol. Again, elevation, icing, and immobility are powerful tools for the reduction of swelling and pain. The following are key points to remember during initial management of a patient with a sprain:

1. Educate the patient appropriately, starting right in the ER. Some sprains may take longer to heal than the corresponding fracture. Many fractures heal reliably within 6 to 8 weeks, whereas some ligament injuries may require up to 3 or 4 months before they can be vigorously stressed.

2. The swelling and ecchymosis that accompany an ankle sprain, for example, can be quite spectacular. Many patients develop a large purple bruise on both sides of the ankle (even if only the lateral side is sprained). This bruise may slowly diffuse like an oil slick, proximally and distally, so that even 2 weeks later, the patient's toes may have a bluish-purple discoloration. Patients commonly call back to the ER several days after their injury, noting nervously that "my toes are turning purple and I'm worried about the circulation." Although every complaint related to blood flow should be considered carefully, toe discoloration in this injury is often nothing more than the usual bruising that results from diffusion of the sprain hematoma.

3. Swelling tends to persist for many months after a sprain and may even persist indefinitely to some degree. This is especially true for the proximal interphalangeal joint of the finger, where a small amount of residual scarring or swelling is noticeable because there is no muscle or bulky soft-tissue plane to hide these changes.

4. Patients also tend to underestimate the potential rehabilitation requirements of a sprained joint. They often express great relief that no fracture has been found and then expect their sprained ankle to be normal in a few days or so. Although a mild ankle sprain may require little attention after several weeks of symptomatic care, a sprained finger can require intensive, supervised hand therapy to facilitate full recovery. As previously noted, the proximal interphalangeal joint is particularly susceptible to irrevocable stiffness because of the anatomy of the joint capsule, volar plate, and collateral ligaments. It helps to instill in the patient a healthy respect for the sprained finger by achieving early motion and establishing a formal routine of daily stretching to accelerate recovery.

Definitive Management

Nonsurgical Management

Type I and II sprains are almost always treated nonoperatively. The ligament ends are connected to their anatomic attachment site. Consequently, immobilization and symptomatic care, as noted in the previous section, will allow healing. Full recovery may depend on a rehabilitation program focusing on strengthening and regaining mobility of the joint that may have been compromised by an initial period of immobility.

Some type III sprains do not require operation. The real issue is whether the ligament is close enough to its anatomic insertion site to yield normal mechanics when healed. This implies also that the joint involved is held immobile during the healing period; otherwise, the ligament presumably will heal out of position. Many surgeons choose not to operate on a type III medial collateral ligament sprain of the knee as long as it is an isolated injury. If, however, other structures of the knee are injured and create additional joint instability or require early mobilization, surgical anchoring of the medial collateral ligament may be indicated so that the ligament can withstand stress during the healing period.

Surgical Management

Occasionally, patients sustain repeated episodes of spraining the same joint. In these cases, each successive sprain episode increases the likelihood of reinjuring the joint, because some residual laxity remains after each injury. These patients may be better served by an operation to tighten the affected soft tissues and thereby make the affected joint less likely to be sprained. Such ligament reconstruction procedures are more likely to be required in athletes. In any situation, these are elective operations that usually follow attempts at treating the "sprain-prone" individual conservatively.

Type III sprains may require surgery, especially if the ligament detaches in such a way that it is not near its original insertion site. An example of this situation occurs at the thumb metacarpophalangeal joint. Injury to the ulnar collateral ligament commonly results from a fall while skiing ("skier's thumb," also called "game-keeper's thumb"). If the ligament detaches completely from its distal insertion on the thumb proximal phalanx, it can become entrapped behind the adductor pollicis muscle's aponeurosis. This is called a *Stener lesion* (Fig. 10–1). The ligament is physically blocked from contacting its native attachment site and will result in permanent laxity of the thumb metacarpophalangeal joint. Consequently, surgery is required to tuck the ligament back underneath the adductor aponeurosis and anchor it back to the proximal phalanx.

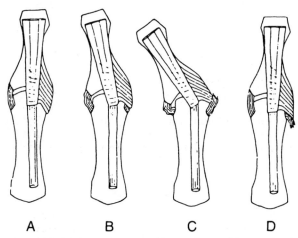

A   B   C   D

Figure 10–1. Demonstration of how a "Stener" lesion develops in gamekeeper's thumb. *(A)* The normal anatomy, with the adductor aponeurosis covering the ulnar collateral ligament. *(B)* Stretching of the metacarpophalangeal joint starts to stress the ligament, which becomes uncovered as the aponeurosis stretches too. *(C)* Maximal stress causes the ligament to fail, with the aponeurosis stretched as well. *(D)* As the joint rebounds to a normal position following injury, the aponeurosis recoils underneath the ulnar collateral ligament, preventing the ligament from resuming normal proximity to its original insertion site at the base of the proximal phalanx. (From Stener, B: Displacement of the ruptured ulnar collateral ligament of the metacarpophalangeal joint of the thumb: A clinical and anatomical study. J Bone Joint Surg 44B:869–879, 1962, p 872, with permission.)

Pediatric Considerations

Children may represent diagnostic dilemmas because a ligament injury can be difficult to differentiate from a nondisplaced (Salter I) growth-plate fracture. The Salter I fracture (see Chapter 7) will not appear as an obvious abnormality on x-rays, nor will a sprain. The physical exam may help distinguish between the two possibilities, because although the growth-plate and ligament attachment sites are usually close to each other, they typically occupy specifically different locations and can be differentiated by careful palpation. Again, knowledge of anatomy makes your job easier.

In general terms, the ligament attachment strength is stronger than that of the growth plate in children, and most children sustain a Salter I injury before the ligament fails. Therefore, the growth-plate injury may be as common or more common than the comparable ligament sprain, but the exact pathology depends on the specific mechanism and circumstances of injury. Fortunately, the distinction between a sprain and Salter I fracture is usually just an academic one, because treatment for either problem is generally the same: RICE and immobilization for a month or so.

TENDON INJURIES

Common Large Tendons

Closed tendon disruptions usually result from sudden excessive load applied to the musculotendinous unit, with failure occurring either within the tendon's substance or at its insertion into bone. Examples of common large-tendon ruptures are those of the patellar tendon, quadriceps tendon, distal biceps tendon (at the elbow), and Achilles tendon.

Peculiarly, these four tendons can rupture spontaneously in healthy individuals from apparently minor trauma. Certainly, the presence of systemic disease, such as diabetes, cancer, or a rheumatologic condition, may be a predisposing factor, but many times no such soft-tissue "weakening" condition may be present. For example, distal biceps tendon ruptures are most common in middle-aged, healthy men, and the precipitating trauma is often minimal (e.g., lifting a heavy book).

Patients usually present immediately if their lower extremity is involved, because they are not able to walk normally. Ruptures of upper-extremity tendons, such as the biceps and triceps, may not be painful enough to provoke medical evaluation right away. The patient may present a few days after the injury, when it is obvious that function has been altered.

Physical exam of large-tendon injuries reveals swelling, tenderness, and often bruising over the site of rupture. *Test the tendon's function because this will be the critical determining test as to the musculotendinous unit's continuity.* For a suspected quadriceps or patellar tendon rupture, ask the patient to perform a straight-leg raise. If the knee extensor mechanism is disrupted, this will be impossible. You can distinguish between a quadriceps and patellar tendon lesion by palpating for a defect proximal or distal to the patella.

Achilles tendon continuity can be examined with a *Thompson's test:*

1. Have the patient lie prone.
2. Bend the knee so that the leg is vertical.
3. Squeeze the calf.

The test result is positive when squeezing the calf does not produce plantar flexion of the ankle. This means that the tendon is ruptured.

Palpation and inspection of the muscle contour are also helpful in assessing upper-extremity ruptures. If the triceps is ruptured, a palpable defect will be present at the posterior elbow. If the distal biceps is ruptured, comparison of the injured antecubital fossa with the opposite side will show that on the affected side, the biceps tendon is absent (it retracts proximally into the arm). This absence can be accentuated by having the patient perform resisted elbow flexion. Furthermore, the biceps muscle tends to look "bunched up" proximally.

Long Head of the Biceps

Rupture of the long head of the biceps is different from that of the other lesions discussed so far for two reasons:

1. The reason for its failure is usually due to osteoarthritis or rotator cuff disease in the shoulder. That is, it less commonly fails in patients with normal shoulder mechanics. The long head of the biceps is subject to attritional wear when the rotator cuff has torn or if osteoarthritic spurs are present near the tendon pathway.

2. Rupture of this tendon does not usually mandate any surgical repair, because the short biceps head (originating from the coracoid process) is still intact. Patients present with pain and ecchymosis about the shoulder of a few days' duration, but ultimately supportive care is all that is required. Function is rarely altered, and therefore treatment is nonoperative. The only residual is an altered contour of the biceps muscle, which will bunch up distally in the arm, giving the patient the classic "Popeye" look. It is difficult, however, to justify any surgical intervention just to change the arm's appearance.

Imaging as an Aid to Diagnosis

As with any injury, plain x-rays constitute part of the usual evaluation plan. In the case of a major tendon rupture, x-rays should be scrutinized for osteochondral fractures or avulsion fragments.

Patellar Rupture

Some patellar tendon ruptures occur with a "sleeve" fracture in which a portion of the patella is pulled off with the tendon. This sleeve of bone is visible on x-ray and is a reliable clue that the patellar tendon has failed.

Knee Extensor Rupture

X-rays are particularly helpful with knee extensor mechanism disruptions, because the patella tends to displace in the direction opposite to that of the tendon rupture. If the quadriceps tendon has failed, the patella will appear relatively distal to its normal position as seen on a lateral x-ray. This low-riding position is referred to as "patella baja." If the patellar tendon ruptures, the patella will become displaced proximally by the intact quadriceps mechanism, and the "patella alta" position is seen on a lateral x-ray.

Magnetic Resonance Imaging

In some rare circumstances, it may be difficult to reliably determine whether a tendon has ruptured. There may be enough swelling or tenderness on physical exam that some doubt may remain about whether the tendon is completely ruptured or perhaps just partially torn. In these cases, magnetic resonance imaging of the affected area may be helpful in making this determination because this test usually can provide excellent soft-tissue detail and accurate information regarding tendon continuity. It is an expensive test, however, and is not routinely ordered unless the physical exam and plain films are inconclusive.

Treatment

Nonsurgical Management

Emergency room management for major closed tendon ruptures is symptomatic. Although operative repair is usually preferred for quadriceps, patellar, Achilles, and distal biceps ruptures, surgery is not required immediately. From your perspective as the orthopaedic consultant in the ER setting, *a bulky dressing with a splint to immobilize the affected joint is standard.* In the lower extremity, non–weight-bearing status (with crutches) is also helpful, as is ice and elevation. Inform patients that they should follow up with the attending orthopaedic surgeon within 1 or 2 days, because although surgical repair is not an emergency, it is far easier to accomplish within the first 5 days or so after injury rather than 2 weeks later.

As previously noted, rupture of the long head of the biceps from its proximal origin at the shoulder is best managed nonoperatively and usually is more significant as a sign of other underlying shoulder pathology, such as rotator cuff failure or osteoarthritis.

Surgical Management

Surgical repair of the quadriceps and patellar tendons is generally mandatory if near-normal ambulation is expected.

Surgical repair of the Achilles tendon is slightly more controversial, because cast immobilization with the foot plantar-flexed will allow the tendon to heal adequately. Some evidence suggests, however, that surgical repair may reduce the likelihood of future tendon rerupture, and the complication rate of surgical repair is low enough to make operative intervention the preferred protocol for many orthopaedists.

Operative repair of distal biceps tendon ruptures is also the usual recommendation because it restores strength and endurance of forearm supination and elbow flexion. However, if the injury is more than a few weeks old, it is very difficult to advance the biceps muscle distally enough to reach its insertion site because the muscle becomes very contracted.

2
PART

*The Orthopaedic
Inpatient Floor*

11
CHAPTER

Preoperative Assessment

HISTORY

Evaluation of a patient for elective surgery is not much different from the assessment described for patients with trauma (see Chap. 1). A good history and physical exam are essential, and the details must be documented carefully. Keep in mind that an organized and focused evaluation should be concise and that most orthopaedic assessments can be written on one or two sides of a page.

Chief Complaint

The history typically starts with the chief complaint (usually using some of the patient's own words) and then a summary of the patient's history relevant to that complaint (also sometimes called the *history of present illness [HPI]*). This part is written as a narrative and is typically three or four sentences long.

Get as much information as possible in these few sentences without having to write a five-paragraph essay. For example, the patient's age, race, gender, hand dominance, and occupation should be contained within the first sentence. Also, ask the patient what worsens the symptoms and what seems to help. Previous diagnostic testing and treatment modalities should also be elicited.

You should be able to create a logical explanation why surgery is now being undertaken.

Medical History

The rest of the patient history should document critical details of the patient's medical background, such as the following:

- Medications being taken
- Allergies
- Prior surgical history
- Substance usage (tobacco, alcohol, caffeine, and illegal substances)
- Other relevant issues, such as coagulation problems and anesthetic history

Focus carefully on allergies, looking not only for medication interactions, but also for latex- or iodine-related problems. There is a growing awareness of patients who are allergic to proteins in latex and natural rubber products, and these patients can respond to the operating room environment with life-threatening anaphylaxis, because many operating room items contain latex (e.g., gloves, drapes, drains). Patients who state they are allergic to shellfish should be considered as possibly allergic to iodine-related medications and contrast media. Remember that allergies, bleeding problems, and anesthesia problems (e.g., malignant hyperthermia, difficult airway) are areas that are easy to overlook and can occasionally produce significant, even life-threatening problems in the operating room. Ironically, it is usually a simple matter to just ask the patient about these issues. Once the "at-risk" individual is identified, adjustments can be made in management that allow surgery to safely proceed.

An overview of the patient's medical and surgical history is relevant because you should be on the lookout for any major medical problems that may influence the outcome of surgery. For example, history of heart attack, stroke, cancer, or infection should be clearly delineated before an operation.

PHYSICAL EXAM

The following are standard elements of a physical exam for a preoperative patient:

1. Include a brief, standard review of the head and chest. It is worthwhile to check neck motion, listen to the heart and lungs, and check for carotid bruits in older patients.
2. Focus on the area to be operated on. The orthopaedic exam can begin with simple inspection, which can identify any visible deformity, skin abnormality, or swelling. Additional key points include range of motion, motor strength, sensibility, joint stability, and any tenderness to exam. It is often worthwhile to document these attributes for the normal side because this provides a nice comparison that highlights the abnormal findings on the affected side.
3. Check for any rashes, blisters, pimples, lacerations, or swelling, which may greatly increase the likelihood of developing a postoperative wound infection and should therefore be carefully noted. The skin surrounding the area of anticipated incision must be normal.
4. Listen to the lungs, and if the patient has a cold, carefully document how long and how severe the patient's cold has been. (The presence of a respiratory illness is another issue that can result in the cancellation of surgery.) If the patient has a cold, contact the anesthesia service. If a general anesthetic has been planned, it may be decided either to use a different method (if possible) or postpone surgery altogether until the "flu" resolves.
5. Although this may seem trivial, identify the side that is to undergo surgery. Make sure that in your written notes "Right" or "Left" is clearly indicated. It may be best to spell this designation out in capital letters, because a simple "R" or "L" can easily be confused, especially if the letter is circled sloppily.
6. *Clearly* write the patient's name, date, and time of exam at the top of your record.

After the physical exam, note the findings of any relevant imaging studies and then summarize your work with a simple "Assessment and Plan" statement. Sign your work at the bottom. Table 11–1 is a sample history and physical exam for a patient scheduled to undergo total hip arthroplasty.

INFORMED CONSENT

Every person who has surgery must undergo the process of informed consent. The attending orthopaedic surgeon is ultimately responsible for the surgery and is the person who should primarily secure consent from the patient. However, house staff are occasionally involved in this discussion. At the least, a good understanding of the informed consent process will add to your clinical skills base.

Purpose and Key Elements

The main purpose of informed consent is twofold: (1) that the patient has some general understanding of the proposed surgery, and (2) that the patient formally gives the physician permission to perform the operation.

Most hospitals have a special form that must be signed by the patient and surgeon in order for the patient to proceed to the operating room itself. You may occasionally see patients stuck in the preoperative "holding area" because the consent form has not been completed or is lost.

The process of signing the consent form itself is simply a paperwork chore. Although it is a good screening tool to make sure informed consent has been addressed, the real consent process is better addressed by a candid discussion between patient and surgeon. How this discussion occurs is a bedside mannerism that each surgeon will choose individually. Gone are the days when it is acceptable to pat the patient on the head and say, "Everything will be fine, don't you worry."

The *three key elements* of informed consent relate to a discussion of surgical risks or complications, the potential benefits of surgery, and the alternative treatments available, including nonoperative choices. (Although it is possible to scare patients out of wanting

Table 11–1. ORTHOPAEDIC HISTORY AND PHYSICAL

History

Patient: John Doe	1/10/99, 8 AM
Chief complaint:	RIGHT hip pain
HPI:	This patient is a 68-year-old, right-hand–dominant, white male retired electrical contractor with a 6-yr history of progressively worsening RIGHT hip pain. He has undergone prolonged conservative treatment with nonsteroid anti-inflammatory medication, physical therapy for strengthening, and several steroid injections. Currently, his pain is severe enough to make playing golf impossible, and he has trouble walking more than one block. Within the past 3 mo, his hip also hurts at night. No history of radiating pain to the foot. No history of trauma. No numbness or tingling in the right leg.
Past surgical history:	Hernia repair, age 19 Appendectomy, age 35
Past medical history:	Hypertension
Current medications:	Aldomet, Zocor, Advil
Allergies:	Penicillin (hives)
Substances:	Tobacco: None Alcohol: 3 beers/wk Caffeine: 2 cups coffee/day Other: None
Bleeding history:	None
Anesthetic history:	Unremarkable
Review of systems:	Viral upper respiratory syndrome resolved 4 wk ago Otherwise negative

(Continued)

Table 11–1. (*Continued*)

Physical

White male in no acute distress	
Vital signs:	Resp 20, BP 130/75, P 82
Height: 5′10″	Weight: 210 lb
Head and neck:	No obvious deformities
	Normal neck motion without tenderness
	No carotid bruits
Chest:	Lungs clear in all fields
Heart:	Regular rhythm, no audible irregularities
Abdomen:	Soft, nontender
	Normal, active bowel sounds
Back:	No abnormal curvatures
	Nontender to percussion
RIGHT hip:	Skin: normal appearance, no discoloration, no swelling
Range of motion:	Flexion: 45 degrees, painful
	External rotation: 10 degrees, very painful
	Internal rotation: 20 degrees
	Abduction: 20 degrees, painful
	Motor: Sciatic nerve and all branches, normal to foot
	Sensibility: All dermatomes in lower extremity intact
	Vascular: 2+ pulse at dorsalis pedis and posterior tibialis
Left hip:	Skin, motor, sensibility, and vascular exams normal
Range of motion:	Flexion: 90 degrees
	External rotation: 70 degrees
	Internal rotation: 30 degrees
	Abduction: 50 degrees

Imaging

Plain x-rays from last month: Severe joint space narrowing and osteophyte formation, RIGHT HIP

Assessment and Plan

RIGHT HIP osteoarthritis, chronic. Failed prolonged conservative treatment. Plan for RIGHT total hip arthroplasty.

surgery by discussing potential operative complications, it is critical to have this discussion.)

Review Risks and Complications

Review the likelihood of each problem, so that a reasonable decision can be made. For example, the infection rate after uncomplicated, primary total hip arthroplasty has been reported to be approximately 1 percent or less. Most patients will realize that such an infection rate is low, and if they have disabling arthritic pain and have tried all other options, surgery will likely be beneficial. However, be sure to involve the patient in the decision making, because many orthopaedic operations are elective and the patient rightfully should have some information on which to base an intelligent decision. Complications of surgery can be divided into two major groups. *General complications* relate to problems that can arise from almost any operation, such as infection; bleeding; nerve, artery, or tendon damage; wound-healing problems; and unattractive scarring. *Problem-specific complications* refer to special risks that are peculiar to the patient's condition. For example:

- Dislocation of the hip after hip arthroplasty is a special risk.
- Sciatic nerve injury after hip arthroplasty for old congenital dislocation is also a special risk.
- Fracture surgery requiring internal fixation may be complicated by nonunion of the fracture or hardware failure.

Fundamentally, the discussion of special risks should focus on how the surgery might fail to achieve the expected results as well as on what subsequent problems might develop if the original condition does not respond.

Review Potential Benefits

The potential benefits of surgery should also be discussed. For example, in managing an open fracture, operative care is mandatory and the potential benefits of infection control would be a key point in explaining to a patient why surgery should be undertaken.

Review Alternative Treatments

Alternative treatment modalities should be reviewed to add some perspective to the patient's apparent choices and reduce the likelihood that a patient may later (postoperatively) feel that he or she didn't have other options presented to him or her. Although the surgeon can certainly indicate his or her preferred management recommendation, the patient should be an active participant in deciding upon a specific treatment course, especially for elective conditions.

The Process of Obtaining Consent

Although the process of obtaining consent may sound daunting, the key determinant is the doctor-patient relationship. Make sure your patients understand what reasonable results are possible with the operation, what could go wrong, and what other choices exist besides surgery. A candid and sincere discussion with your patient will usually make the consent process quite natural.

Beware, however, of patients who even indirectly request a "guarantee." *Never* suggest that you can guarantee anything. Even the simplest operation can produce major problems. Remember that there is virtually no condition that cannot be made worse by surgery. Also be wary of patients who are impatient to sign a consent form without really discussing the operation and its potential complications. These are the very patients who will be the most upset by any subsequent trouble that develops, screaming the whole time that "no one ever told me this could happen."

Whenever you are faced with a lack of understanding, poor communication, or just plain-old peculiar behavior by the patient, be extra cautious. Review the treatment options many times, don't rush the patient to any conclusions, and proceed with your informed consent process more carefully than ever. Be ready to cancel the procedure if you have any doubt about the patient's understanding.

The Consent Form

Although the consent form must be signed by the patient and surgeon, the form itself is less important than the discussion process. Therefore, most attending physicians will have a dictated summary of this discussion in their office notes, because this dialogue typically occurs in the office. For patients undergoing less elective procedures (trauma), a notation should be made in their hospital record that reflects the informed consent process. Just be aware that having the patient sign a consent form is the minimum adequate documentation. More detailed notes should be available either in the hospital chart or the office record. The least satisfactory method of consent occurs when the patient signs the form in the operating room holding area. Many times the patient will have already received some sedation or narcotic, thereby making the consent interaction potentially meaningless. Furthermore, the informed consent process should be mediated by the attending orthopaedic surgeon, who is familiar with the patient and his or her treatment course. As a medical student or resident you may help complete paperwork, but it is poor form for you to be the primary authority for securing consent, because often you will be meeting the patient for the first time on the day of surgery.

Sample Consent Form

The following is an example of an informed consent notation for a patient planning to undergo a carpal tunnel release. This type of note is written in the office record before the surgery date or possibly written in the hospital chart. Remember that hospital-chart consent notes are usually more appropriate for patients who are admitted to the hospital and then undergo surgery before discharge (e.g., patients with trauma).

> I have discussed in detail the different treatment alternatives for carpal tunnel syndrome with Mrs. Doe. Conservative measures, such as splinting, anti-inflammatory medications, steroid injection, and activity modification have not been effective, and her symptoms are worsening. I have recommended carpal tunnel release surgery as an option that may have better efficacy in reducing her symptoms and helping to prevent worsening muscle weakness. The risks and benefits of surgery have been discussed at length. Risks of surgery have been noted to be inclusive of (but not limited to) infection, bleeding, nerve, artery, or tendon damage, wound-healing problems, hypersensitivity, scarring, and failure to relieve

her current signs and symptoms. In particular, I noted to Mrs. Doe that the length and completeness of recovery from surgery are variable and she may require up to a full year to experience maximal improvement, and that maximal improvement from surgery may not mean complete resolution of her complaints. Furthermore, she understands that numbness and weakness may be permanent residuals despite surgical intervention, especially in view of her advanced physical findings and severely abnormal nerve conduction test. She also understands that it is possible that surgical intervention may prove to yield no improvement at all.

All these issues were discussed in detail, and all of Mrs. Doe's questions were answered. The technical details of surgery, postoperative immobilization protocol, and possible need for postoperative hand therapy were also reviewed. In particular, she knows that her outcome may be critically dependent on her meticulous participation with a postoperative hand therapy program, which could require significant time and effort contributions on her part. She understands the treatment options and risks of surgery and wishes to proceed with carpal tunnel release.

PREOPERATIVE ORDERS AND LAB TESTS

In the mid-1980s, almost every patient was admitted to the hospital the day before surgery. Sunday afternoon was a big event because droves of patients would arrive at the hospital scheduled for surgery on Monday or Tuesday. Medical students and residents had to "work up" these new admissions, which meant writing a history and physical and then specifying the preoperative admission orders. Even when I wasn't on call for the weekend, I frequently had to come in on a Sunday afternoon to help the on-call house staff with the paperwork for our usual dozen or so orthopaedic admissions.

Now, however, most patients are admitted on the same day as their surgery, usually just a few hours before they are taken to the operating room. The preoperative lab tests, as well as other details of the presurgical routine, have been arranged by the attending surgeon's office ahead of time. Therefore, the house staff have much less involvement in organizing preoperative care for elective admissions. Nonetheless, many patients still rely on you to arrange their trip to the operating room. Inpatients who need orthopaedic care represent one such population. The most common "preop" situation that you will arrange is for a patient admitted through the emergency room.

The main practical focus for the house officer who is writing preoperative orders is to make sure that the patient's surgery is not canceled on a technicality. Certainly, if the preoperative workup reveals an abnormal lab test or some other issue that demonstrates increased risk, cancellation is appropriate. In fact, the basic concept behind the preoperative workup is to make sure that no hidden risk factors jeopardize the patient's safety. But your mission is to avoid cancellation "on a technicality."

There are several simple, avoidable "technical" reasons why a patient's surgery would be canceled.

1. **Eating or drinking before surgery:** A patient cannot eat or drink for 6 to 8 hours before surgery, because a full or partially full stomach increases the risk of aspiration into the lungs. Even if a regional or local anesthetic is anticipated, most anesthesiologists prefer that patients remain NPO (nothing per os) for the required time. Whether it's really 6 or 8 hours preop depends on the anesthesiologist and the situation. Patients often forget this rule or treat it casually. Be aware that many anesthesiologists will cancel an elective operation if the patient admits he ate just one cornflake. Patients are sometimes allowed to take their regular medication with a sip of water on the morning of surgery. However, with respect to food items, nothing by mouth means *nothing*.

2. **Omission of certain basic lab test results from the chart:** This requirement varies depending on the patient's age, the type of surgery, and the particular rules of the specific institution. In the mid-1980s, it was routine to order just about every available blood test for every patient. Now, because of cost scrutiny, many fewer lab tests are ordered routinely. However, just about every patient undergoing surgery in a main operating room must have a complete blood

count. Patients older than a certain age (often 45 or 50) also require an electrocardiogram. Patients with cardiac, renal, or diabetic problems usually require more complicated blood chemistry panels. For procedures that may involve significant blood loss, coagulation tests (prothrombin time, partial thromboplastin time, platelet count, and bleeding time) are appropriate, as well as consideration of arranging blood donors (if the patient doesn't donate his or her own blood ahead of time). Patients undergoing a major joint arthroplasty often have a preoperative urinalysis to make sure that they do not have an ongoing urinary tract infection at the time of surgery. There is no simple formula as to what lab tests to order, because the proper screening depends on the patient's medical history, the operation itself, and the "house rules."

Of some help is the fact that for most patients older than 50 or those who have any complexity to their medical history, their internist or family doctor is usually the one responsible for conferring "medical clearance." This includes performing a complete history and physical exam and ordering whatever tests are necessary to ensure that the patient's condition is optimized for the planned surgery.

3. **Problems with medication before surgery:** Patients with diabetes should check with their internist or endocrinologist as to how much insulin they should take on the morning of surgery. It may be necessary to take some medication on the day of surgery by mouth, so again, check with the internist as to what's necessary. Preoperative sedation is no longer routinely ordered; if any is necessary, the anesthesiologist will often administer it in the holding area. Some procedures, such as total joint arthroplasty, require antibiotics to be given 30 to 60 minutes before surgery. Check with the orthopaedic attending physician about specific preferences.

4. **Lack of a completed history and physical exam and a signed consent form on the chart.**

Table 11–2 is a handy checklist summarizing the major preoperative orders. Note that many items (indicated with an asterisk) apply only if required by the patient's age, medical history, or operative complexity.

Table 11–2. PREOPERATIVE CHECKLIST

1. NPO after midnight (or 8 h before surgery)
2. History and physical on chart
3. Completed informed consent on chart
4. Medical clearance note on chart (if necessary)
5. Labs
   a. CBC
   b. ECG (if age >45)
   c. Blood chemistries*
   d. Coagulation profile*
   e. Urinalysis*
   f. Chest x-ray*
   g. Type and screen for blood transfusion*
   h. Sickle cell prep (for African-Americans)*
6. Medications
   a. Patient to take own meds with a sip of water (check with both the anesthesiologist and internist)*
   b. Antibiotics: administer IVPB on call to OR*

IVPB = intravenous piggyback ; OR = operating room.
*Only if required by the patient's age, medical history, or operative complexity.

THE HOLDING AREA

The holding area is where patients wait just before being rolled into the operating room. This is often where the anesthesiologist first meets the patient. Frequently, the IV lines are started here, and some initial sedation is given (after consent form is signed!). Family members are usually not allowed in this area unless the patient is a child.

The holding area affords you, as part of the surgical team, the opportunity to confirm two critical details before entering the operating room: the patient's identity and the part of the body to undergo surgery. This may sound ridiculously obvious, but be warned that it is not. Furthermore, a mistake on either of these issues is catastrophic.

Patient and Part Identification

Adhere to the following guidelines for identification of the patient and the part that will undergo surgery.

1. **Check the patient's identity.** Talk to the patient
   and make sure the chart, name band, and any other
   paperwork all say the same thing.
2. **Identify the part that will undergo surgery.** This
   is a trickier issue. If the patient is being treated for
   a fracture, it's usually obvious which side (right or
   left) is the operative side. However, even in the patient with trauma, it can be easy to make a mistake.
   For example, some patients present with *bilateral
   injuries*. In fact, sometimes another injury may not
   even have been diagnosed, adding the potential for
   significant confusion in the operating room. For example, you thought you were going to débride a
   right-hand dog bite; then in the operating room you
   discover that *both* hands have draining puncture
   wounds. What does the consent form say? The patient is heavily sedated and when questioned will
   only hum show tunes. Shouldn't you treat both
   hands? Or, was the left-hand injury not even related
   to the current trauma? The best answer is not to ever
   get into this situation.

   Even more treacherous is when the patient is having an elective procedure. You will have no obvious
   external landmarks to distinguish between the right
   or left carpal tunnel as the symptomatic one.
   Arthroscopy and total joint arthroplasty are two
   other common procedures for which the operative
   side must be clearly determined before the patient
   is in the operating room. Remember that when under
   general anesthesia, a patient cannot tell you which
   side is the correct one. It is frighteningly easy for
   someone to be taken to the operating room, be put
   to sleep, have the wrong side prepped (because the
   operating room schedule is wrong), become fully
   draped, and then have the surgeon walk in and start
   work on the wrong extremity. In fact, you cannot
   easily tell a right thigh from a left thigh if the patient
   is fully draped and turned on his or her side.

   The problem with identifying the proper side for
   surgery is that it seems like such a trivial and obvious
   issue. However, the attending orthopaedic surgeon
   is ultimately responsible. You need to get into the
   habit of making side identification a part of your
   normal routine. "Routine" is the key word, because

rigorous, unyielding routine will be your best defense against making a side identity mistake. Your interaction with the patient in the holding area should follow a similar routine that then extends into the operating room. Introduce yourself to the patient and make sure that he or she is the right person to be operated on. Ask the patient if he or she has any questions about the surgery. Then ask what operation is being performed and on which part of the body. I routinely then mark the correct part with an indelible surgical marker. Every single patient gets the same treatment. No patient goes back to the operating room without being identified by me and without my mark on the correct part. You may choose to develop your own system, but a system of some sort must be present.

The American Academy of Orthopaedic Surgeons has promoted a campaign called "Sign Your Site" that encourages attending surgeons to mark the correct extremity by signing their initials on it. The AAOS campaign recommends using an indelible marker (so that the prep process cannot wash off the markings). It also suggests signing the site close to where the anticipated incision will be made so that the identifying marks will be obvious even after the patient is fully draped for surgery. Surgeons should then proceed with making the incision only if they see their initials close by, confirming the proper extremity.

3. **Verify** that what the patient identifies as the correct side corresponds with what the operating room staff and chart indicate, using several different methods, such as the patient's record (which I bring to every operation), the x-rays, the consent form, and the operating room schedule. These four methods of notation must correspond with what the patient just indicated in the holding area. Be aware that *the operating room schedule is notoriously incorrect,* and to make matters worse, it is usually used by the operating room staff as the exclusive method of identifying the correct side. Check the chart, x-rays, and consent form. Ask the patient directly. Mark the side.

Verifying the correct side is the ultimate responsibility of the attending physician, but you cannot start learning this routine too soon.

In the operating room, hang the appropriate films on a view box. These should indicate clearly the correct side. Before the side is prepped, personally recheck that the side being washed has your mark (e.g., your initials) on it.

12
CHAPTER

Postoperative Care

After surgery is completed, you are responsible for writing a specific set of orders and discharge instructions. This chapter reviews common features of the postoperative care plan for orthopaedic patients and also discusses standard "discharge instructions" that each patient should receive before going home. The postoperative note and operative dictation are reviewed at length in Chapter 16.

INPATIENT CARE

The postoperative orders constitute the guidelines by which the nursing and ancillary staff administer care. Although writing these orders may seem like a lot of busy work, you will be setting the critical parameters that dictate the management of each patient in the crucial days after surgery. Before we get into specific details, a few general rules should be noted.

1. **Write clearly:** Many mistakes in care delivery that adversely affect patients relate to medication errors, and often the problem originates from sloppy handwriting. Although physicians are associated with poor penmanship of legendary proportions, there is no excuse for illegible writing when it may affect patient safety. Write your orders clearly, even if it takes much more time.

2. **Note the time and date of your orders:** Most medical record departments will recall your charts if you

skip this detail anyway, but the real issue is accurate, complete documentation of care. Furthermore, if any questions arise after the fact about your care plan or what was ordered, you will stand to benefit greatly if the date and time of your orders are clearly registered.

3. **Be as complete as possible.** You should be able to write a complete set of postoperative orders that will give the nursing staff no reason to page anyone to ask for additional specifications. For example, you will remember to write a prescription for a standard sleeping medication after you are called several times in the middle of the night to add it. What if routine narcotics make the patient a little nauseated? Anticipate this common occurrence by writing for prochlorperazine (Compazine) or promethazine (Phenergan). You may have written for a variety of narcotic pain medications, but did you include plain old acetaminophen? Many patients benefit from this for mild pain management, but the nurses will have to page someone to get the order approved. The main concept here is that by anticipating the routine course of your patient, you can write a complete order set that will make the nurses' job easier and result in fewer midnight pages requesting approval for routine items.

4. **Anticipate the patient's discharge** early, literally right from the recovery room. For hip fracture patients, for example, hospital discharge often requires an assessment of the patient's home environment and independent living skills. Family members are frequently anxious about sending their loved one home too early or may be concerned that the patient cannot live alone for the first few weeks of recovery. Usually, the hospital's social service is consulted for "discharge planning" to help make these decisions. Consult the social service people early. In fact, it is wise to write for a social service consult right in your postoperative orders. The same is true for any physical therapy or other ancillary support. The sooner you order the consult, the more likely the desired consultant will show up in a timely fashion and not delay your patient's progression to discharge day.

Specific Inpatient Postoperative Orders

Until you develop your own specific preferences for writing postoperative orders, the following list can be used as a starting point because it contains a nucleus of basic orders. Specific additional orders must be added to this list depending on the operation. This basic set of orders is the one I was taught as a surgical intern and is relatively arbitrary. There are many satisfactory ways to organize postoperative orders; after you gain some experience, you may come up with a better system of your own.

A helpful mnemonic is ADC-VANDALISM. This stands for:

A—Admit
D—Diagnosis
C—Condition
V—Vitals
A—Allergies
N—Notify service
D—Diet
A—Activity
L—Labs
I—Intravenous
S—Surgical site care
M—Meds

A indicates that you must designate where the patient is to be *admitted* from the recovery room. This is typically to the orthopaedic floor.

D for *diagnosis* reminds you to write (as a separate line) the patient's diagnosis, primarily to inform the nursing staff (and anyone else caring for the patient) of the primary surgical issue. For example, for a patient undergoing total hip replacement surgery, the diagnosis would read, "S/P Total Hip Arthroplasty for Osteoarthritis."

C for *condition* specifies the status of the patient after surgery. Although I have rarely seen this line written as anything other than "Stable," writing for the condition of the patient is a time-honored tradition and helps make you consider for a moment the patient's medical stability.

V for *vital signs* reminds you to write an order for the patient's vital signs. Specify how frequently they should be taken and that this data must be recorded in the chart. It is also common to include a "circulation, motor, and sensory (CMS) status check" or check of the neurovascular status of the limb with the vital signs.

A represents documentation of the patient's *allergies*. This is placed as an order because it is so important that the nursing staff is aware of any potential contraindicated medications. Writing the letters "NKDA" indicates that the patient has no known drug allergies.

N for *notify* refers to telling the nurses when to page you for a problem. This order is typically written relative to vital signs and changes in the neurovascular status. Common notification parameters are as follows: T>101.5°F, BP>140/90 or <100/60 mm Hg, a resp >24 or <12, and P>120 or <60. Any change in the extremity's neurovascular status or pain unresponsive to adequate medication also should prompt a call.

D for *diet* is usually written as "general," or even better, "advance to general as tolerated." This gives the nurses some latitude in feeding patients, because many people are nauseated for the first 24 hours after anesthesia. Diabetic patients may require more specific diet orders.

A for *activity* represents a critical issue for orthopaedic patients. Can your total hip replacement patient put full weight on the leg that has been operated on right away? This will depend on the type of replacement performed and the surgeon's preference. Remember that some spinal surgery patients may not even be allowed out of bed initially. Specifically, ask your attending physician about the patient's activity status so that you can write the appropriate order. This is also a good time to write a consult order for physical therapy, because it may take 1 or 2 days for the physical therapists to actually commence the rehabilitation program. If the therapists know the patient just had surgery, they can already meet their prospective new client and plan a timely schedule.

L for *labs* refers to the lab tests that need to be ordered. Actually, for orthopaedic patients, very few lab tests need to be routinely ordered. Hemoglobin and coagulation studies are most commonly ordered, usually for patients undergoing hip or knee arthroplasty.

I for *IV lines* indicates that you must write an order for the care of existing IV lines. Usually, fluids through these lines can be tapered to zero as the patient tolerates a general diet. You may not want to remove the line completely, however, until all medication given by an IV route (usually antibiotics) has been administered. Therefore, it is common to write an order that indicates changing the IV line to a "heplock," which should remain in place until all IV medications have been given as ordered.

S for *surgical site* reminds you to write an order directing care for the wound and any drains that may be present. Drain output should be charted every shift, and wounds are kept dry. If the surgical site is in the distal extremity, you may add an order to elevate the affected part to help with pain relief and swelling reduction.

M for *medications* may involve a long list of drugs, including antibiotics, pain medications, antinausea agents, a "sleeper" (sedative to aid sleep), anticoagulation medicines, stool softeners, vitamins, and any other medication that the patient may ordinarily take.

The basic mnemonic, ADC-VANDALISM, will help get you started, but it is by no means complete. A complete set of orders will depend on the exact nature of the surgery and the complexity of the patient's underlying medical status.

The following are additional issues that need to be addressed in orthopaedic patients with more complicated conditions:

1. **Foley catheter:** Chart the patient's output. Furthermore, before removing the catheter, have the nurses send a clean-catch urine specimen for culture.
2. **Anticoagulation protocol:** In patients undergoing pelvic or lower-extremity surgery, many surgeons routinely order specific measures intended to reduce the incidence of deep vein thrombosis. Some of these measures may be pharmaceutical (aspirin, heparin, warfarin [Coumadin], etc.). and some measures may be mechanical (sequential compression boots, foot pumps, elastic stockings). Remember, also, that certain medications require daily coagulation studies to monitor their effect.
3. **Imaging studies:** Some surgeons routinely order screening studies such as venous Doppler imaging. This topic is highly controversial, and it is probably

best to ask your attending physician directly what measures are preferred for each patient.

A Set of Sample Orders

Remember that you will adjust medication doses and IV fluid rates based on the patient's weight and medical status. The following is a set of basic orders for a hypothetical knee replacement patient.

8/12/98 2:00 PM

1. Admit to 4 South Orthopaedics.
2. Diagnosis: S/P Total Knee Arthroplasty for Osteoarthritis.
3. Condition: Stable.
4. Vitals: q4h x 4, then q shift. CMS checks with vitals. Record vitals and CMS checks.
5. Allergies: NKDA.
6. Notify service if T>101.5° F, BP>140/90 or <100/60, P>120 or <60, RR>24 or <12, urine output <30 mL/h, or any change in CMS checks.
7. Diet: Advance to general as tolerated.
8. Activity: Up to chair in AM. May be full weight bearing on operated leg with walker. Consult physical therapy to see patient ASAP for above activity.
9. Labs: CBC q AM x 2. PT/PTT q AM while in hospital.
10. Finish OR bottle at 75 mL/h and start D5.45NS + 20 mEq KCl at same rate. Change to heplock when PO intake tolerated well.
11. Surgical site: Keep wound dry and elevate knee. Maintain knee in CPM machine as set by orthopaedic service.
12. Meds:

    a. Morphine: 4–6 mg IM q3h PRN pain.
    b. Phenergan: 25 mg IM q3h PRN pain or nausea.
    c. Tylenol with codeine: 1 to 2 tabs PO q4h PRN pain.
    d. Tylenol: plain, 650–1000 mg PO q4h PRN pain.
    e. Ancef: 1 g IVPB q8 h × 48 hours.
    f. Restoril: 15 mg PO qhs PRN insomnia.
    g. Colace: 100 mg PO bid

   h. Multivitamin: 1 tab PO qd.
   i. Coumadin: Call service daily for dose after
      morning lab result is back.

OUTPATIENT CARE

   Writing postoperative orders for outpatient surgery
is intrinsically simpler because the patient's care period
is only a few hours long rather than a few days. Furthermore, the surgery tends to be more limited in scope,
and the patients are healthier.
   Nonetheless, the ADC-VANDALISM method of organizing your orders still applies. Two additional issues
need to be addressed almost immediately when you are
writing for the care of a "same-day-discharge" patient.

1. Specify what bandages or supplies the patient should
   take on discharge. For example, patients undergoing
   hand surgery often use a sling to keep their hand
   elevated and supported during the first few days
   postoperatively.
2. Specify discharge criteria. A common discharge order reads as follows: "Patient may be discharged if
   PO is tolerated well, patient has voided, oral pain
   medication is sufficient, and patient understands follow-up care plan."

DISCHARGE INSTRUCTIONS

   Every patient who leaves the hospital, whether after a
few hours or a week, must have written instructions that
specify recommendations for follow-up and posthospi-
tal care. The underlying principle for these discharge instructions is quality of care. Furthermore, most hospitals
have a policy that absolutely requires a physician to sign
off on written discharge instructions, so expect the
nurses to page you if the instructions are not completed
by the time the patient is ready to go home.
   Most surgical units have a "Discharge Instruction"
form that lists specific items that you are to fill out.
However, you may not always be able to find the form
and it is helpful to be familiar with the key elements of
discharge recommendations. The following list summa-

rizes common issues for orthopaedic patients who are leaving the hospital environment after surgery:

1. Indicate exactly with whom the patient should follow up by listing the surgeon's name, office address, and phone number.

2. Indicate when the patient should be seen in the office. Ask the attending if you are not sure. Also, write clearly that the patient should call the office within 24 hours to arrange the first postoperative appointment. This is a particularly helpful point for your attending physician, because many patients tend to believe that they automatically have a postoperative appointment scheduled and can simply walk into the office anytime. This often makes for an unnecessarily hectic office day.

3. List the medications that the patient should take. This may include pain medication, antibiotics, and anticoagulants. Do not write the doses as if you are writing a prescription, because most patients will not be able to decipher medical shorthand.

4. Note any special care requirements. Helpful comments include keeping the bandages dry, elevating the distal extremity for pain control, and moving unaffected joints.

5. Indicate that the patient should come to the emergency room (ER), call the office, or page the attending surgeon if any serious problems arise. List phone numbers. The definition of a serious problem should then be noted to include severe, unremitting pain, worsening swelling not responsive to elevation, wound drainage, temperature higher than 101.5°F, or progressive numbness, tingling, or coldness distal to the operative site.

You should note that discharge instructions should also be written out for patients leaving the ER after care for an orthopaedic condition. Although filling this information out for every ER and surgical patient may seem like a chore, it is a matter of safety and patient education that cannot be skipped.

MORE COMMENTS ABOUT POSTOPERATIVE ORDERS

Two more common issues about postoperative orders deserve mention:

1. Transferring a patient to the medical service
2. Transferring a patient out of the intensive care unit (ICU).

As you sit in the recovery room after operating on a patient for a broken hip, for example, the temptation is to "transfer the patient to the medical service." One reason this may be appealing is because the medical service will have to write all the orders. Resist this temptation, because it bears false hope.

The best reason to admit or transfer an orthopaedic patient to the medical service is because his or her medical problems (e.g., brittle diabetes, heart disease, renal failure) greatly overshadow the complexity of the orthopaedic problem. In borderline cases, however, you are probably better off with the patient on the orthopaedic service. That is, it's better for the patient because the orthopaedic floor nurses know better how to manage orthopaedic problems. The advantage from your perspective is that you receive far fewer pages and experience much less frustration if the patient is in the orthopaedic area. A patient on the medical service still requires that you make rounds just as frequently (and usually requires walking farther in the hospital).

Traction devices, casts, and orthopaedic bandages are seen as complex foreign objects by nonsurgical nurses and in the end become much more labor intensive for you. Do not be fooled into attempting to transfer one of your patients to the medical service because the workload seems potentially easier. It will actually be harder and you may be doing the patient a disservice. Base such decisions solely on where the patient's more complex problems will receive the best attention.

Another smaller issue arises with orthopaedic patients who are residing in the intensive care unit. When the patient is ready to be transferred out of the ICU (to the orthopaedic floor), you must write a set of "transfer orders" that are identical with a complete list of postoperative orders. Although this may seem to be duplicate work, do not hesitate or skimp to create this new set of orders. The floor nurses must have complete and detailed information to care for this patient. Just because the individual was in the ICU for a few days doesn't mean that the floor nurses know any more about that patient than if he or she had come directly from the recovery room. For reasons that are not completely clear, some house staff continue to believe that transfer orders from the ICU are unnecessary or redundant. Do not make this mistake. In fact, as soon as you suspect one of your ICU patients may be ready for transfer, write the order set and tell the ICU nurses that your paperwork is ready. The ICU nurses will appreciate your organization and promptness, and your patient will be transferred out smoothly.

13

Special Postoperative Issues

Management of orthopaedic inpatients requires that you can diagnose and treat a variety of postoperative and postinjury situations that are predictable. This section reviews several major categories, focusing on problem recognition and the basics of immediate intervention.

ANESTHETIC PROBLEMS

Administration of anesthesia is often responsible for a variety of patient complaints postoperatively—some trivial and some potentially more serious. Perhaps the most basic principle in deciphering these problems is to *ask the anesthesia staff for help.* Although this advice sounds obvious, it is often ignored. Whereas the medical record will provide helpful information such as fluid volume administered, estimated blood loss, and so on, do not hesitate to ask the anesthesiologists for help. They often have special experience and insight that easily solves your clinical problem. Furthermore, patients prefer increased contact with the anesthesiologist, and therefore, their involvement has a positive effect on patient public relations. Remember, surgery is a team event, and it will be of great advantage to you, both in and out of the operating room, to maintain a good rapport with the anesthesia staff.

General Anesthesia

Common immediate complaints after general anesthesia relate to the upper airway manipulation required for endotracheal intubation. The first logical step, therefore, is to be certain whether the patient was actually intubated. Be aware that for some shorter procedures, mask ventilation or use of a laryngeal mask anesthesia (LMA)–type tube does not involve tracheal manipulation.

Upper airway manipulation can produce a variety of relatively minor complications, such as the following:

1. Loosened or chipped teeth or dental work and lacerated or swollen lips sometimes result from difficult intubations (often in patients with short necks or limited neck extension). You can usually reassure patients that swollen or cut lips will resolve in a few days with no significant residual effects. Symptomatic care, such as ice, often helps. Any significant dental damage should be assessed by dental professionals, but get the anesthesiologists involved first. Sore throat is perhaps the most common postintubation complaint. This almost always resolves by itself over several days. Throat lozenges, acetaminophen, and cold food often serve as the best symptomatic measures.

2. Blurred vision may be medication-related, although it can also result from a corneal abrasion or other minor trauma to the eye that occurs while the patient is asleep. As with dental problems, contact the anesthesia service first for an opinion.

3. Pulmonary compromise is a common problem after general anesthesia, especially in elderly patients or in anyone who has even slight preexisting pulmonary risk factors, such as asthma, emphysema, or cigarette smoking. Atelectasis, or collapse of the basilar segments of the lungs, is usually temporary, but it is the most common reason why patients manifest a low-grade fever after surgery (see later in this chapter

regarding fever). Patients should be strongly encouraged to get out of bed and breathe deeply, because these activities help reexpand the lower lung segments. Use of incentive spirometry can be helpful to force patients to breathe deeply on an hourly basis.

Any serious cardiac or pulmonary issues are usually related to the patient's preoperative medical history and the length and scope of the operation. Problems such as pneumonia, heart failure, or pulmonary edema should be addressed by the appropriate services, usually anesthesia and medicine. Careful documentation of the patient's fluid status (input and output) during and after surgery can be critical in determining proper management.

Regional Anesthesia

The most common types of regional anesthesia for orthopaedic procedures include spinals, Bier blocks, and axillary blocks. These anesthetic methods are excellent choices for outpatient procedures because the patient's cognition is less affected than with general anesthesia.

Although these methods of anesthesia have an excellent safety record, you should be aware of a few possible problems:

1. **Local toxicity:** It is always possible for local anesthetic toxicity to occur, especially in patients who may have arbitrarily low thresholds to local agents. Although this is rare, suspect this in patients who complain of ringing in their ears or in those who demonstrate any evidence of cardiac or neurologic symptoms after a regional block. Get the anesthesia service involved immediately.

2. **Prolonged numbness:** Another common issue relates to how quickly the block wears off. The motor and sensory blockade of a Bier block (IV administration of local anesthetic into the upper extremity) reliably wears off within 20 to 30 minutes after the tourniquets are released. However, spinal and axillary blocks can last for several hours, depending on what agent was used. Sometimes the nursing staff may call you noting that the patient cannot move

the toes or fingers yet, or that the patient is "still numb." First, check the anesthesia record and identify what type of block was administered. Many times, the patient's numbness or weakness just reflects persistence of the anesthetic. Be aware, however, that most blocks wear off a few hours after the procedure, so if the neurovascular changes are persistent, further work-up is warranted.

2. **Bruising:** Use of a tourniquet is common for many upper- and lower-extremity procedures, and sometimes long tourniquet times produce bruising underneath the tourniquet. It is even possible to inadvertently get iodine paint solution underneath the tourniquet and subsequently cause burns in sensitive individuals as the tourniquet squeezes the painted skin. Many surgeons prefer to wrap a plastic drape around the lower margin of the tourniquet to prevent scrub solution from seeping underneath.

3. **Paresthesia:** Tourniquet pressure also occasionally accounts for postoperative paresthesias, especially in obese patients. This numbness or tingling is usually diffuse and radiates distally from the tourniquet site. It usually is not severe enough to manifest as a complete motor block. Once you rule out other more serious causes, simple observation is all that is required; the paresthesias will reliably resolve spontaneously.

NEUROVASCULAR CHANGES

Patient Assessment

Every patient who sustains orthopaedic trauma or undergoes an operation requires neurovascular monitoring of the operative extremity. This is often referred to as "CMS checks," with CMS referring to *c*irculation, *m*otor, and *s*ensory status. In patients with trauma, the CMS status should be well documented during the initial physical assessment so that a baseline is established for later comparison. Most patients undergoing elective surgery have normal neurovascular findings in the affected extremity, although don't assume this is so. It is just as important to document sensory and motor function preoperatively so that if any changes occur after surgery, you will know whether action is required or not.

For example, patients who have sustained a stroke or who have diabetes may not have normal motor and sensory function before their total knee arthroplasty. If their peroneal-nerve motor function is weak in the recovery room, how do you know if this is due to operative trauma to the nerve or whether it is the patient's normal baseline?

When you have documented the patient's preoperative status carefully, have the extremity checked at intervals postoperatively. It is good practice to examine the patient yourself in the recovery room (or once the anesthetic as worn off) so that you are confident that the affected region has returned to preexisting neurovascular function. Write orders for the nursing staff to perform CMS checks at intervals, usually with vital signs. Also write for the CMS checks to be recorded, so that you can quickly see an overview of the patient's time course of recovery and identify if and when any problems started.

Neurovascular checks after surgery or trauma are used to identify two types of problems.

1. **Single-event injury to nerves or blood vessels:** For example, after total hip arthroplasty, it's good to document that the sciatic nerve is working. Correction of a severe valgus deformity through knee arthroplasty may stretch the peroneal nerve. In the recovery room, you should be able to document (through the physical exam) that these nerves are working, thereby establishing that the operative procedure has not compromised them in any way.
2. **Progressive compromise, due to such factors as swelling, bleeding, compression, or ischemia:** An example is bleeding that occurs from a segmental tibial fracture that produces a compartment syndrome. This type of problem can be identified through a careful, frequent physical exam. For high-risk situations, such as long-bone fractures, spinal cord and pelvic injuries, and crushing trauma, it is often appropriate to write orders for CMS checks every 1 or 2 hours for the first postinjury day to make sure that progressive deterioration of function is not overlooked. Whereas use of pulse oximetry can be

helpful to assess blood oxygenation to the distal extremity, do not become too dependent on machinery. A direct physical exam is by far the best way to monitor the CMS status.

When the nursing staff pages you because they're concerned about a patient's CMS status, you must take them seriously every time. It is true that, in a large proportion of these cases, the patient is fine, but you cannot afford to miss the one real case of progressive neurovascular compromise. Not only can such compromise produce severe permanent impairment for the patient, but also such situations are usually avoidable if caught and treated.

Rereading the section on compartment syndrome (see Chap. 1) might be helpful at this time. Postoperative and postinjury patients should be monitored with compartment syndrome principles in mind. Patients who are experiencing pain that is crescendo in nature, out of proportion to their injury or surgery scope, or unresponsive to seemingly adequate pain medication must be carefully assessed. This is the kind of pain that ischemia can produce. Again, remember that pain thresholds are quite subjective and individualized, and many patients may be just anxious or undermedicated. However, do not presume that this is the answer until you have fully assessed the patient yourself.

Intervention

When the nursing staff calls and says that your patient with ankle fracture is writhing in pain and having foot numbness, the first thing you should do is examine the patient yourself right away. Meticulously assess motor and sensory function and make a judgment as to why the pain is severe. The following are possible reasons for the continuing pain:

- If the neurovascular status is normal, perhaps the pain medication should be increased or changed.
- The patient's foot may not have been elevated enough after surgery.
- The dressing or cast may be too tight and must be loosened. (This problem can result in compartment syndrome.)

Whatever you recommend (perhaps all of the above), the key principle is close follow-up of the patient's response. If you make a minor change and the patient immediately improves, fine. But if no improvement in comfort or function occurs within 30 minutes, continue to pursue the issue until resolution. Never tell the nurse just to increase the pain medication and "we'll see how he does in the morning." Good nurses will continue to bother you until the patient is better, and it is your responsibility to make sure the neurovascular status is maintained at baseline.

Pain Patterns

Pain is a difficult complaint to assess. Patients demonstrate a wide variety of pain responses, some of which will be colored by individual personalities, expectations, and anxiety. In general, however, most traumatic and surgical orthopaedic pain responds to elevation, immobilization, and routine pain medication.

Ominous pain patterns include a "crescendo" pathway, in which the pain seems to worsen steadily with time, regardless of the treatment administered. This type of pain is characteristic of ischemia and must be thoroughly investigated. Even though each patient's response to medication may be slightly different, most orthopaedic discomfort can be managed with routine narcotic use. Most postoperative conditions can be managed easily with intramuscular injections of morphine or meperidine (Demerol) for 1 or 2 days. Patients typically can then be switched to oral medication such as hydrocodone or acetaminophen with codeine.

Be wary of any patient who seems to fall outside the usual medication requirements. Do not assume that such individuals either are substance abusers or are just being difficult; either conclusion should be the last one you draw. First, you need to rule out absolutely issues such as nerve compression, compartment syndrome, and other causes of local ischemia.

Neurovascular Changes

If you find that the neurovascular status is altered significantly, you must immediately effect intervention (and notify your attending surgeon). Intervention usually requires loosening or even complete removal of all casts, bandages, or traction devices. Sometimes the answer will be simple, such as a brace pushing too hard against the lateral knee causing peroneal nerve dysfunction. Removal of the brace and gently bending the knee usually relieves pain immediately followed later by motor recovery.

The postoperative dressing and splint applied after ankle fracture surgery may need to be loosened to allow for swelling. Remember that not only can a cast be too tight, but the underlying cast padding may need to be released as well. Ace bandages have a tendency to bunch up as the patient moves around in bed. In some circumstances, they can produce a tourniquet effect. (Note: When applying an Ace or elastic bandage, always wrap loosely and start distally [toes or hand] and work proximally. An Ace bandage that is wrapped from proximal to distal has a tendency to partially unravel and act as a limb tourniquet.) In the case of reimplantation surgery or free tissue transfers, postoperative swelling may so tighten the finger or graft that skin stitch removal at the bedside is necessary to relieve pressure and reestablish improved blood flow.

If you cannot resolve the patient's symptoms of increased pain or paresthesias or if the patient seems to have a new deficit in motor function or vascularity, continue to aggressively investigate until the problem has been resolved or you have a definitive diagnosis. It is sometimes necessary to remove all the bandages completely before accurate assessment of the limb can be performed.

Any patient whom you suspect might have a compartment syndrome should have compartment pressures checked and documented. Even if it later turns out that the patient was just anxious and undermedicated, the worst problem of removing the cast or checking pressures is just inconvenience, whereas the mistake of missing a compartment syndrome or nerve injury can be catastrophic.

Feel free to contact the attending if you are concerned about a patient. Certainly call the attending if you check compartment pressures, even if the pressures are normal. Most attendings will want to know about any potential problems early in their development.

When discussing a particular patient on the phone with nursing staff, you may hear someone say, "He is in a lot of pain, but his pulses are normal." For some reason, the peripheral pulses get a lot of focus in assessing patients after trauma or surgery, when, in fact, the distal pulse exam may be misleading. A full-blown compartment syndrome can be present with normal distal pulses, so the presence of normal arterial pulses is not any guarantee of safety. Certainly, if the pulses are absent when they were previously present, you must immediately investigate. However, unless you are monitoring a patient who underwent peripheral vascular surgery, a pulse exam may be of minor importance compared with a sensory, motor, and soft-tissue tension exam.

If you are in the process of assessing a patient and elevation of the limb with a slightly loosened dressing seems to have helped, don't forget to reassess the patient in another hour or so. The most consistent feature of a nerve or vascular problem is that the problem persists and worsens progressively. Although it may initially seem to be labor intensive, it is good practice to reexamine the patient yourself every 1 or 2 hours if you have any doubt as to the patient's response to intervention. Although the nursing staff may document CMS checks frequently, *you* also should examine any patient that seems to be unusual or problematic. Do not make the mistake of treating pain and swelling too casually if it persists or is out of proportion to the usual recovery course. Remember, patients who have undergone limb-saving emergency fasciotomy for compartment syndrome usually began the whole ordeal by first complaining to someone (you) that their leg or arm "really hurts" or that the pain medication "just doesn't seem to work." Most orthopaedic residents, by the time they are done with residency, can recount at least one story in which their personal involvement with assessing a patient in pain caught an incipient compartment syndrome and ultimately led to intervention (e.g., fasciotomy) that saved the limb.

FAT EMBOLISM

In some patients with long-bone fractures, fat emboli can cause severe pulmonary compromise through both mechanical and chemical pathways. Intravascular emboli can block perfusion and produce a ventilation-perfusion ($\dot{V}/\dot{Q}$) mismatch. Furthermore, the breakdown products of fat particles include free fatty acids that can have a toxic effect on the alveolar lining cells. Pulmonary edema and hemorrhage can result and become severe enough to be life-threatening.

Clinical Manifestations and Treatment

Fat embolism syndrome is not understood enough to be completely preventable, but be aware of its presentation so that early treatment can be initiated. Most patients manifest the clinical syndrome of fat emboli within 12 to 48 hours of injury. Shortness of breath and anxiety are two early findings, followed by low-grade fever and increased heart rate.

The classic precipitating injury is a femoral shaft fracture, but fat embolism can also occur from any event that produces intravascular dissemination of fat particles. For example, some cases are believed to result from total knee arthroplasty procedures in which intramedullary femoral guide-rod placement pressurizes the femoral canal and forces marrow fat particles into the bloodstream.

Neurologic status may decline progressively until the patient is disoriented or even comatose. A classic physical finding after the first few postinjury days is the presence of petechiae on the chest wall, axilla, base of the neck, or conjunctivae.

Lab assessment should include arterial blood gas measurement, which typically demonstrates significant hypoxemia. Chest x-rays may demonstrate a progressively worsening "snowstorm-type" picture, due to increasingly severe pulmonary infiltrates.

Treatment is supportive and may require respiratory support in an intensive care setting. Administration of oxygen is the cornerstone of care, supplemented possibly with steroids and antibiotics, depending upon the physician's preferences and the individual circumstances.

BLEEDING

Blood loss is not typically a major problem in orthopaedic surgery because many procedures are amenable
to use of a tourniquet. Furthermore, most hip and shoulder procedures follow predictable planes of dissection,
and blood loss is usually minimal even though it is
not possible to apply a tourniquet. Most intraoperative
bleeding occurs from exposed bone surfaces that arise
either from fracture or intentional preparation by the
surgeon. The following are situations calling for particular attention to bleeding:

1. **Trauma:** In trauma patients, the most significant
   blood loss often occurs before they get to the operating room. That is, fractures have the capacity to
   bleed vigorously, and long bones such as the femur
   can account for several units of blood loss into the
   thigh. Pelvic fractures can bleed enough to become
   life-threatening (see Chap. 3). It is important to
   check the patient's hemoglobin level before surgery
   to get some idea of their general condition. Remember that the fluid status can influence the lab result,
   so dehydrated patients, for example, will have a hemoglobin that is artificially elevated.
2. **Major spine or joint procedures or significant
   trauma:** It is worthwhile to check the patient's hemoglobin level daily for a few days after major spinal or
   joint surgery or in patients with significant trauma.
   Once their blood count stabilizes or starts to rise,
   additional testing is probably not necessary. In cases
   of massive blood loss, elderly patients, or patients
   with significant preexisting cardiac disease, it may
   be necessary to involve the internal medicine service
   to carefully manage the patient's blood and fluid
   status.
3. **Drains** are typically inserted in orthopaedic wounds
   that have the potential to bleed postoperatively. The
   drain's primary function is to prevent formation of a
   large hematoma by allowing the excess accumulated
   blood to escape. Drain output should be recorded
   every 8 hours. Although most drains can usually be
   removed after 1 or 2 days because their output is low,
   keep track of these numbers. Occasionally patients
   manifest significant or steady output, which may be

a sign that they have persistent surgical bleeding in the operative site or that a coagulopathy exists.

4. **History of bleeding or anticoagulant use:** A coagulation history should be obtained from every patient. Ask about "easy bruising" or any family history of bleeding problems. Be sure to note what medication is being taken, especially anticoagulants such as warfarin (Coumadin) or aspirin. Before major procedures, coagulation lab work is often checked routinely, and in patients with any predisposing history or medication use, partial thromboplastin, prothrombin times, and bleeding should definitely be measured.

Many patients who are planning elective joint replacement donate 1 or 2 units of their own blood before surgery and use that blood preferentially if they need a postoperative transfusion. Although a hemoglobin level of 10 g used to be a rough guideline below which transfusion was considered, with the current concern about transmissible disease, many internists and orthopaedists now prefer to withhold transfusion unless the hemoglobin level drops below 9 g or even lower. These judgments also depend on whether the patients have their own blood available and on the patient's general medical status (sicker individuals may not be able to tolerate a lower hemoglobin). It is a good idea to check with your attending physician before ordering a transfusion, because in most situations the decision-making process is very case-specific.

THROMBOSIS

Thromboembolic disease is a controversial topic because the science governing clot formation is complicated and not completely understood. Unfortunately, however, deep venous thrombosis (DVT) is a common orthopaedic complication. In fact, it has been estimated that a DVT is likely to occur in 60 percent of patients with hip or knee arthroplasty if no prophylactic measures are used. Of these patients, 10 to 15 percent are likely to develop a pulmonary embolism, and 1 to 3 percent will sustain a fatal pulmonary embolism.

A common risk factor within the orthopaedic world is pelvic or hip surgery. Furthermore, traumatic conditions as well as elective surgery can place the patient at risk. Hip fracture patients who are not treated with some form of prophylaxis will experience a 3 to 12 percent mortality rate due to thrombotic events.

Risk Groups

Surgical patients can be categorized into different thrombosis risk groups depending on the number of many risk factors present. The specific list of risk factors is long and seems to include almost every imaginable condition. However, a core group of conditions is considered to make up the classic "precondition" for thrombosis formation:

- Previous history of thromboembolism
- Pelvic or hip surgery
- Obesity (>120 percent ideal body weight)
- Stroke or spinal cord injury
- Malignancy
- Older age
- Prolonged surgery (>2 hours) or prolonged immobilization
- Multiple trauma

Some authors characterize a high-risk patient as one who has three or more of these factors. Prophylaxis measures have been stratified, based on which risk category is present. For example, a moderate-risk patient (two risk factors present) may be managed with elastic stockings and low-dose heparin injections. A high-risk patient may be managed with sequential compression boots and administration of warfarin. Remember that the exact recommendations (and the specific assessment of individual thrombosis risk) are heavily influenced by the details of each particular patient and surgeon preference.

Part of the reason why treating physicians tend to vary in their management or prophylaxis of thromboembolic disease is that many times the attending physician is strongly influenced by the last bad clinical experience. Occasionally, a clot (and even a subsequent pulmonary embolus) develops in a supposedly low-risk (or no-risk) patient. Almost every attending physician can relate a story about how a symptomatic clot formed after an ankle or elbow procedure. The apparent randomness of this bad event precipitates a tendency for "anecdotal medicine" that borders on superstition more than science. Usually, upon scrutiny, these low-risk patients actually do have some risk factors such as obesity or prior history, although this may not be evident at the time of presentation. Furthermore, there are undoubtedly patients in whom no clear risk factors are present despite the formation of a clot. Unfortunately, some portion of thrombosis science still remains a mystery.

Prophylaxis

A major area of controversy centers on methods of preventing thrombosis and their respective efficacy. The two main categories of prevention include anticoagulants and mechanical methods:

1. **Anticoagulants:** Anticoagulant drugs include warfarin, heparin, aspirin, dextran, and low-molecular-weight heparin. Key issues that characterize choice of drugs include route of administration and likely bleeding complications. For example, heparin must be administered either IV or as an injection, whereas warfarin can be taken orally. The effect of heparin is easy to reverse and wears off within 4 hours, whereas the anticoagulant effects of warfarin can take 3 days to diminish. The best drug would be one that can be taken orally, wears off quickly, produces little risk of postoperative bleeding, and effectively prevents DVT.

2. **Mechanical methods:** Elastic compression stockings, sequential compression boots, and foot pumps are examples of currently used modalities to fight thromboembolic disease. Similar to the different drugs, some of the mechanical modalities are more appealing than others based on convenience, patient toleration, and purported efficacy.

The exact method that you use for prophylaxis of your postoperative patients will depend specifically on the preference of the attending surgeon. In fact, because the science and clinical realities of clotting are not yet completely understood and because clot formation can represent a potentially fatal complication in some cases, a certain degree of superstition tends to creep into the particular management protocol that individual practitioners use. Therefore, ask your attending physician in every case whether thrombosis prophylaxis is necessary and, if so, what method should be ordered. Almost no two attendings use the exact same protocol, and many people prefer to mix the use of both drug and mechanical modalities.

Clinical Presentation and Diagnostic Work-up

The two basic clinical presentations of thrombosis are that of a DVT and that of a pulmonary embolus. Remember that in both situations, the clot can be present and remain completely asymptomatic.

The classic DVT presentation is one of calf swelling and pain. Warmth and some redness may also be present, and patients will note that walking or pressure on the calf is painful. It is sometimes possible to palpate firmness near the affected vessels, although generally the entire muscle compartment is soft (in distinction to a compartment syndrome).

Patients with *pulmonary embolus* may present in a variety of ways, ranging from mild shortness of breath to sudden cardiac collapse and death. Sometimes the initial findings may be nothing more than presence of a low-grade fever. Any pulmonary symptoms or unexplained fever in a surgical patient should be taken very seriously. Furthermore, hypoxia may initially present as gradual or mild confusion. A patient with postoperative hip fracture with the onset of new mental disorientation, for example, should be thoroughly assessed for possible thrombosis.

Diagnostic work-up depends on the degree of clinical presentation. If a pulmonary embolus is suspected, it is usually evaluated with a $\dot{V}/\dot{Q}$ scan, which is a nuclear medicine study that can identify those areas of the lung that have diminished perfusion (blood clot blocks blood flow) relative to the usual ventilation. A more accurate (and also much more invasive) study is pulmonary angiography. The decision to order these tests is often made with the advice of an internal medicine consultant. The most common scenario is that of a patient presenting with shortness of breath, tachycardia, or hypoxia, and a V̇/Q̇ scan is obtained immediately.

For diagnosis of DVT, Doppler ultrasonography is standard. This test is noninvasive, easy to perform, and reliable as long as experienced personnel administer and interpret the test. The gold standard in terms of accuracy is a venogram, but similar to pulmonary angiography, this test requires intravascular dye administration and has some associated risk.

Many orthopaedic surgeons routinely obtain an ultrasound study of the legs in postoperative arthroplasty or patients with fracture if they have undergone procedures involving pelvic or lower extremity surgery. Although some authors have challenged the cost-efficiency of obtaining these "screening" ultrasound studies, many orthopaedists feel safer checking their pelvis and hip surgical patients just before discharge from the hospital. Check with your attending physician to find out the preferable protocol.

Treatment

Treatment of established thrombosis depends on the following :

- Where the clot is located
- Under what circumstances the clot formed
- Whether the patient is clinically compromised by the clot

Most pulmonary emboli are thought to arise from clots in the femoral system, so many surgeons do very little to actively treat an asymptomatic clot located in the calf vein system. If a calf DVT is symptomatic or if a more proximal clot has been identified, treatment with warfarin for 3 months is commonly recommended. Furthermore, as soon as the diagnosis is made, IV heparin is typically started along with the oral warfarin because it takes several days for the warfarin to achieve a therapeutic effect.

Depending on your attending physician's preference and the hospital environment, you may occasionally find it helpful to consult the medicine service for advice. In fact, because there is so much variation as to how clots are treated (and for how long), it is a good idea to contact the attending surgeon as soon as the diagnosis is made.

Treatment for an established pulmonary embolism focuses first on supporting the patient's oxygenation and immediate clinical well-being. The anticoagulation protocol is similar to that previously described, although warfarin is usually administered for at least 6 months. If a clot formed while the patient was already anticoagulated or if the patient cannot tolerate anticoagulation drugs, then placement of a vena cava filter is often recommended.

WOUND INFECTION

It is crucial to identify postoperative infection problems, because early recognition greatly facilitates treatment. Furthermore, many nonorthopaedists believe that the presence of a fever in any postsurgical patient signals a wound infection, and this is in fact infrequently the case.

Only a few bacteria have the ability to produce a wound infection within 24 to 48 hours of surgery, and these include group B streptococcus and *Clostridia* organisms. The most common offending organisms, *Staphylococcus aureus* and *Staphylococcus epidermidis*, usually take 7 to 10 days to produce clinical infection. Therefore, most patients with wound infections do not present the day after surgery, but rather a week or more later. You may not even see many wound infections during the primary hospital stay because even after major procedures such as joint arthroplasty, most patients don't stay in the hospital for more than 4 or 5 days.

Patients with wound infections initially present with classic signs of erythema, swelling, tenderness, and possibly drainage. It may be difficult to identify how deep the process extends. Some dramatic surface findings may indeed represent only a superficial process. And conversely, deep wound infections may not initially produce dramatic superficial skin findings. Deep extension of the infection can be a disaster, threatening whatever implants may be present in the total joint patient, or producing the catastrophe of osteomyelitis. Therefore, any patient with an apparent wound infection must be treated carefully.

If you suspect a wound problem is present, follow these steps:

1. Attempt to culture any drainage that might be present.
2. Send off appropriate lab work, including a white count, sedimentation rate, and blood cultures.
3. Review the patient's temperature record and vital signs since the time of surgery and note any patterns of abnormality.
4. Probe the wound carefully, if possible, to gain some appreciation as to how deep the process extends, but be careful not to incidentally open the wound and cause more contamination or damage than already present.
5. Obtain an x-ray of the area just to make sure that no loosening of arthroplasty components or bone erosions are obvious.

Management of wound infections is a complicated subject, but from a practical standpoint, surgical débridement and antibiotic coverage are two of the standard modalities. Consultation with the infectious disease service can be greatly helpful, and ultimately the work-up and subsequent decision-making process often constitute a team effort.

Wound "Irritation"

Sometimes a surgical wound may look reddened and yet not seem to be infected. Remember that the presence of staples or sutures for more than 10 days sometimes causes skin irritation. If the wound looks mature enough to withstand suture removal, taking out the stitches often resolves this skin irritation immediately. Staples in particular have a tendency to cause skin erythema in some sensitive patients. Note the surgical date so that you don't accidentally remove the sutures too soon and cause the wound to open up. Placing some skin tapes (Steri-strips) over the wound is a good way to maintain a little mechanical stability right after removing sutures.

Drainage

Some patients have clear, yellowish drainage from their wound for up to 2 weeks after surgery. This is more common in obese patients or wounds that are in fatty areas, such as the thigh or buttocks. The drainage usually represents a process of fat necrosis and does not involve infection, but it is smart to culture it anyway. Patients will manifest no other symptoms or signs. The drainage may just be a small amount, or it can be enough to soak dressings on a daily basis. Although such drainage is usually self-limited, it does pose some increased risk of infection and should be minimized, if possible. If the drainage is enough to stain dressings several times a day, many orthopaedists start the patients on antibiotics (oral route if the patient is going home). Increased attention to dressing care and iodine painting of the wound margins with each dressing change are also sometimes recommended until the drainage stops. Perhaps the most effective method in obese patients is to prevent the patient from lying on the wound and getting the patient out of bed. Direct pressure on the wound and shear forces that arise from rolling around in bed frequently prolong serous drainage.

Toxic Shock Syndrome

Toxic shock syndrome is caused most commonly by *S. aureus* colonization. It can be rapidly fatal, and you should be aware of this process because it can occasionally occur in postoperative wounds. Affected patients demonstrate a very high fever, and the wound typically shows some drainage, although the amount may be relatively unimpressive. The drainage should be cultured, looking for staphylococcal organisms. If the process is allowed to progress, the patients will suffer the effects of the bacteria's toxin production, including hypotension, nausea, vomiting, and diarrhea. Ultimately, multiorgan system collapse can occur with an ensuing 7 to 10 percent overall mortality rate.

Treatment of toxic shock syndrome depends on early recognition and immediate wound débridement with appropriate antibiotic administration.

FEVER

The presence of a low-grade fever after surgery is so common that it may be incorrect to presume that it is an abnormality. However, fever may also be the best single indicator of an underlying problem, so it is wise to follow temperature data carefully.

Low-grade fever usually refers to a temperature of less than 101.5°F. It may be helpful to recall the "four W's" of the postoperative fever: *w*ind, *w*ater, *w*ound, and *w*alk.

- *Wind* refers to atelectasis and is usually a problem in patients who have undergone general anesthesia or have preexisting pulmonary compromise. Getting the patients out of bed and use of an incentive spirometer (or respiratory therapy in severe cases) may accelerate the resolution of lower lung segment collapse.

- *Water* refers to a urinary tract infection, which may account for a fever in the first few days postoperatively. Send a urine culture and urinalysis to the lab, and then remove the Foley catheter (if present). Oral antibiotics are usually sufficient in resolving most urinary tract infections.

- *Wound* refers to fever due to wound infection, which was previously discussed.

- *Walk* represents fever due to DVT (thought to be partially caused by immobility and venous stasis). Keep in mind that thrombosis of the proximal femoral veins and pelvic vessels can lead to pulmonary embolus and that occasionally such major thrombosis may present as a fever of unknown origin. Appropriate work-up usually includes internal medicine consultation, laboratory work-up (blood gas measurement and other tests), and relevant imaging studies, such as venous Doppler studies of the lower extremity or $\dot{V}/\dot{Q}$ scanning of the lungs.

Low-grade temperature can also be caused by the presence of hematoma, which is certainly common after surgery. Look for significant swelling (often elliptical in shape) and bruising. Patients who are taking anticoagulant medication or who have coagulopathies are at particular risk for developing a hematoma. Many hematomas can be managed with observation only because they slowly resolve spontaneously. If the wound is compromised by undue tension or drainage, then the hematoma might be better managed by surgical evacuation.

More esoteric causes should be sought in patients with postoperative temperatures higher than 101.5°F. Advanced infection, toxic shock syndrome, substance withdrawal, and sepsis are examples of processes that might produce high fever.

FALLS IN THE HOSPITAL

As in any other institution in which there are many people, accidents occur with some regularity in the hospital. Because of your role as the orthopaedic consultant, you should have some idea of what role you play in the "fall" scenario.

Hospital Personnel

First, it is worthwhile to mention your role in dealing with hospital personnel who are injured on the job. You may be eating breakfast in the cafeteria when someone, either a cafeteria worker or a patient's family member, slips on a wet floor and falls down. It is not unusual for the orthopaedic house staff to be identified and then expected to "do something." Unfortunately, your role is not that of a paramedic, and you must be careful not to worsen the situation. Certainly, you can perform whatever immediate first aid is necessary and reasonable, such as splinting an obviously broken leg or helping someone into a chair. But don't get fooled into providing any definitive advice or treatment without formal assessment. Call security and help facilitate transferring the victim to the emergency room (ER) so that proper medical evaluation can be performed. If the person is trapped in a machine or seriously hurt, rescue professionals may be better suited to extricate and transport him or her. Even if the injury seems relatively minor, it is probably wise to encourage the person to stop by the ER and have the injury reviewed by an ER physician. If you give casual advice without proper assessment, you might do more damage than good, even if your intentions are noble. Just because you might know the person who fell doesn't mean that you can assess the ankle injury without x-rays and a proper physical exam.

Patients

Unfortunately, patients themselves may fall in the hospital, sometimes while walking or trying to get to the bathroom. Occasionally, they fall out of bed. It is smart to treat every such consultation for a "fall" with a formal assessment. It is possible for a patient to have a broken hip from a fall in the hospital and not be diagnosed for several days.

Another common scenario is that "something happens" in physical therapy. That is, after a therapy session, the patient (or therapist) notes that the patient is experiencing more pain than usual or is struggling to catch himself or herself from a "near-fall" experience. If the patient has a significant complaint, it is also wise to treat these episodes as presumptive injuries until proven otherwise.

After any fall scenario, follow these guidelines:

1. Examine the patient carefully after obtaining a good history.
2. Obtain appropriate x-rays (at least AP and lateral films) of the injured area. If the patient underwent an orthopaedic procedure and has implants in place (i.e., total joint components or fracture hardware), compare the postfall x-rays with immediate postoperative films, and note carefully whether anything has changed. Look particularly for loosened screws, bent plates or wires, or movement of joint implants.
3. After you have fully interviewed and examined the patient and reviewed the films, write a detailed note in the chart with the date and time to clearly document a record of events and your findings.

IMPLANT DISLOCATION

Dislocation of an orthopaedic implant is a variation of the fall scenario. Although many patients may dislocate their joint arthroplasty long after surgery and present "de novo" to the ER, other patients actually dislocate their implant during their hospital admission (or even in the recovery room!). The most common situation is the dislocated total hip arthroplasty. Evaluation of the patient proceeds in the following manner:

1. Initially assess the patient through a brief history and physical exam. Find out when the patient's surgery took place, who the surgeon was, and why the patient underwent arthroplasty.
2. Examine the extremity to make sure that neurovascular function is normal.
3. Obtain appropriate films so that you can clearly understand which way the implant dislocated. Although an anteroposterior (AP) film of the hip may show a dislocation most dramatically, you cannot determine whether the implant is dislocated anteriorly or posteriorly without a shoot-through lateral view. As usual, you may need to assist the radiology technician in holding the patient's uninjured leg out of the way to obtain the proper views of the injured side.

Reduction

Once you know which way the dislocation has occurred, the next issue is how to effect a reduction. It may be best at this point to call the attending orthopaedic surgeon and ask how to proceed, because so much personal preference is involved in performing a reduction. For example, if the patient has undergone implantation of complex revision components or has poor bone stock, some attending physicians prefer to perform a reduction under anesthesia with fluoroscopic control. This approach minimizes the possibility of loosening the components or fracturing the femur. On the other hand, if the patient is a disoriented nursing home resident with a simple unipolar implant placed because of previous hip fracture, the attending physician may suggest that you first attempt a simple closed reduction in the ER or hospital room. A simple maneuver, in this situation, may pop the hip back in place without any comorbidity.

If you do attempt to reduce a dislocated hip by yourself, proceed in much the same way as you might for a traumatic dislocation of a normal hip. First, appropriate sedation and traction are required. Then, proceed according to the following guidelines:

1. For the common posterior dislocation, hip flexion and adduction may be initially required to "unlock" the femoral head from the acetabular rim.
2. Then, gradual external rotation, extension, and abduction will bring the head over the rim and back into the socket. Remember that if the patient is not relaxed enough, even the slickest hip maneuver and five people pulling on the leg may never effect reduction because the patient's muscles have a much greater mechanical advantage than you do.
3. Some dislocations are just plain difficult to reduce. If you are struggling a lot, there is no dishonor in calling your attending physician back and asking for advice or help. Actually, that's a sign of a smart house officer.
4. Try to avoid performing the reduction in the patient's room. The softness of the hospital bed and the narrow confines of most hospital rooms prevent you from maintaining good positioning of the patient or of yourself or getting good mechanical purchase of the leg or torso. It is usually safer to transport the patient to a treatment room or even the ER if the environment is not ideal. Certainly if any significant sedation is required, you must have appropriate monitoring (e.g., pulse oximetry, blood pressure). Again, the ER may be the best place.
5. After reduction seems to be accomplished, repeat orthogonal x-rays. Remember that a completely dislocated hip can appear perfectly reduced on a single AP x-ray. *Obtain the AP and lateral films to properly confirm that the joint is back in place.*
6. Document your reduction care with a note in the patient's chart or ER record.

URINARY RETENTION

Postoperative urinary retention is not uncommon, especially in older men after a general or spinal anesthetic. Many older men suffer from benign prostatic hypertrophy anyway, and the administration of an anesthetic makes it difficult to urinate postoperatively. Furthermore, patients are frequently bedridden the first few days after a major procedure, and it is even harder to urinate if the patient is lying down.

Note that more than one male patient has been admitted for hip arthroplasty and wound up staying an extra few days for a prostate evaluation or treatment for a chronic urinary tract infection. With this in mind, specifically ask patients preoperatively about their urinary tract history, both with respect to frequent infections (especially in women) and urinary retention or frequency (particularly in men).

Urinary retention is a problem because it can ultimately damage the urinary system if not treated in a timely fashion; furthermore, it makes the patient very uncomfortable. The following are approaches to relieving the patient's urinary retention:

1. **Mobilization:** The first and simplest method of getting patients to urinate may be just getting them out of bed. Sometimes the sound of a running bathroom faucet also helps them initiate urination more easily.
2. **Catheterization:** It may be necessary to catheterize the patient (or recatheterize, as the case may be). It is reasonable to have a catheter in place to relieve a full bladder, although multiple passes of the catheter or an indwelling catheter for more than 1 or 2 days increases the risk of developing a urinary tract infection (something particularly unsavory in a new postoperative patient with total joint arthroplasty). Therefore, it may be practical to leave a catheter in place for 1 or 2 days after surgery until the patient is ambulatory and, therefore, more likely to get out of bed to urinate. If you have to catheterize a patient for retention, leave the catheter in place overnight and then remove it in the morning, when the patient is more likely to be mobile.

Whenever you remove a catheter, have the nurses send a sample of urine for culture, so that if an infection does develop later, you have a clean-catch sample that will more accurately allow organism identification.

If urinary retention cannot be resolved after 1 or 2 days or requires more than one episode of recatheterization, consult the urology service for help.

THE CONFUSED PATIENT

Occasionally, you will be asked to evaluate a patient who is confused. *The critical issue is whether or not the confusion represents an acute change or whether confusion was present before injury or surgery.* This again places emphasis on carefully obtaining and documenting a history and physical exam.

1. **History:** Many elderly patients who present to the ER appear quite lucid. However, you must actually ask them questions about their current situation to identify whether they are truly oriented. Moreover, the patient's family may also insist that "grandma has always been clear as a bell until she was in the hospital," when in fact "grandma" was barely functioning independently and the hip fracture itself is an omen that she cannot be safely independent any more. An injury and subsequent hospitalization may be just enough to tip the balance of mental clarity. This clarity can often depend on familiar faces and environment, so that a postoperative patient with hip fracture may appear to be totally disoriented. This can be a shock to the family, who insist that grandma has suddenly deteriorated.

2. **Documentation:** Carefully document preoperatively if the patient wasn't too clear on any specific details of time, place, or situation. This will help you properly characterize any confusion later identified as "new."

3. **Clinical assessment:** The issue surrounding new onset of confusion is that mental disorientation is often the main (and sometimes only obvious) sign of hypoxemia. Therefore, rapid onset or worsening confusion must be worked up to identify the source of hypoxemia, such as myocardial infarction, pulmonary embolus, sepsis, stroke, or overmedication. This last factor is particularly common in the hospital environment, because many elderly patients are acutely sensitive to small doses of narcotics and sedatives. Even if the patient was not totally oriented on admission to your service, you must first address major physiological causes of hypoxemia in assessing the confused patient before you assume that

he or she is just reacting poorly to a strange environment.

4. **Laboratory studies:** Immediate work-up of the confused patient includes checking a blood gas or pulse oximetry reading. This important step helps to establish whether the patient has enough oxygen circulating in the bloodstream. Low oxygenation should be aggressively pursued, probably with an ECG, $\dot{V}/\dot{Q}$ scan, and additional studies to identify any central neurologic problems or sepsis. An internal medicine consultation is usually helpful, also.

5. **Medications:** In your initial assessment of the confused patient, review the past 48 hours of medication administration in the written record. It is surprising how many times a little extra narcotic administered in the recovery room or on the first postoperative day may result in decreased respiration, lowered oxygen content, and mental disorientation. Many times a narcotic reversal agent administered IV will improve the patient's outlook within 30 minutes.

Only when a thorough medical and neurologic work-up produces no abnormal findings can you conclude that new onset of confusion does not portend an ominous, underlying physiological disorder. What will help you the most in the middle of the night when a nurse pages you about a disoriented patient unfamiliar to you is the documented admission history and physical exam.

3
PART

The Operating Room

14
CHAPTER

General Principles

The orthopaedic operating room (OR) sustains its own special "culture," defined in part by the specialized equipment used, the special skills of the nurses and support staff, and the complex mechanical nature of the operations performed. Understanding a few special features of this orthopaedic environment will help your learning experience to progress more smoothly.

TEAMWORK

The team concept lies at the heart of the OR culture. The surgeon can function alone no more than a pilot can run a commercial flight by himself. The OR "crew" consists of the surgeon, a scrub nurse, a circulating nurse, an anesthesiologist, usually an anesthesiology assistant (nurse anesthetist or resident), and a surgical assistant (often a resident or student). For the team to function best, everyone must be willing to help out and focus on getting the job done quickly and safely.

The operation itself is only one part of the total project in caring for a surgical patient in the OR. The airplane analogy applies well here also: Flying the plane is only part of the crew's work. Seating the passengers, instructing them about safety, providing food and comfort during flight, preparing them for landing, helping them depart the plane, and cleaning the aircraft to prepare for the next trip are all part of the team's job.

Your willingness to be a team player will greatly increase the respect and responsibility afforded to you by the other "crew" members. A multitude of small tasks can be better accomplished with several sets of helping hands. Wheeling the patient back to the OR works better with two or three people guiding the cart. Getting warm blankets for the patient, padding the patient's bony prominences, getting tourniquet equipment ready, obtaining lead vests for everyone if fluoroscopy is to be used, performing the sterile prep of the surgical area, and hanging appropriate x-rays are just a few things that you can do before surgery begins that will be appreciated by your teammates.

After the operation, be ready to help move the patient back to the cart and help transport him or her to recovery. There should be no task that is "beneath" your status. I have occasionally helped clean the OR table and floors in an effort to help turn the room over more quickly. House officers and medical students who understand the team concept are more likely to be accepted by the staff. Furthermore, most attending physicians view your participation in surgery as something that is earned through your willingness to help with all aspects of patient care, not just with the "fun" parts.

NURSES

Although you may already appreciate the importance of being pleasant and respectful to your coworkers, you will find good interpersonal skills to be especially valuable in the OR. And although you may believe that your behavior in the OR clearly shows unbridled enthusiasm and sincerity, many OR nurses take a dim view of medical students and junior residents—and not without cause. The following are a few tips and suggestions on how to behave in the OR:

1. Most OR nurses have worked for several years in the same environment and have seen scores of house officers come and go. Unfortunately, they have had to work in close quarters with an "occasional" arrogant, underskilled, and condescending character. As you might imagine, the legacy of a few bad apples tends to linger. Keep this in mind.
2. Furthermore, the OR nurses' position within the hospital hierarchy is often inversely related to their functional importance in the operative setting. One of

the worst things you can do is to irritate or demean these critical players. Ask any experienced surgeon; the talent of the scrub and circulating nurses is often why a case goes smoothly.

3. Be careful not to confirm the nurses' negative stereotype of the junior team member. Introduce yourself humbly and try to remember their names right away. Respect the nurses' preferences and speak as politely as possible. Say "thank you" a lot and smile, even if the atmosphere may be a little cold at first. In addition, even if you think your way is better, succumb to their requests on how to stand, sit, scrub the patient, gown yourself, put on your mask, put on your gloves, or any other seemingly minor detail. Chances are the nurses have performed these tasks thousands of times (and with each particular attending), and their way is probably more efficient.

4. Study how the nurses move and handle equipment, and you will learn OR skills quickly. Many new medical students are unable to join the OR team without standing directly in the way of nurses or threatening to contaminate sterile equipment every other minute. However, if the nurses like your attitude, they will quickly teach you all these little "style" points, and your comfort level and self-confidence in the OR will skyrocket.

5. Never condescend or attempt to humiliate anyone, or you may quickly find yourself quite alone in a crowded room. When I was an intern, I saw a particularly egocentric surgeon scolding an experienced scrub nurse to hand over the instruments faster. All afternoon the scrub nurse was slapping instruments into the surgeon's hand, saying "here it is, *doctor*." After the operation was over, I asked the scrub nurse why she kept saying "doctor" with such a peculiar tone. She smiled and said that at this hospital, all the nurses generally referred to the surgeons by name, but when someone simply said "doctor," they really meant "asshole."

CHECKING THE PATIENT'S IDENTITY AND OPERATIVE SIDE

A habit that you should adopt quickly is verifying that the patient you are about to operate on is the correct person. Check the chart, the patient's ID bracelet, and then actually introduce yourself and call the patient by his or her last name. The job of checking identity is one that the attending surgeon and several nurses will undertake as well. Even though all this duplication of effort may sound silly, a mistake of identity is one that cannot be prevented too carefully. (These very important checks are covered also in Chapter 11.)

Checking that the proper side of the patient's body is undergoing surgery can be even trickier. Don't doubt that a limb can be marked, prepped, draped, verified by a sedated patient, and then undergo the correct operation, except on the wrong extremity! I recommend a systematic approach to both the patient's identity and limb identification. In fact, the American Academy of Orthopaedic Surgeons (AAOS) recently issued guidelines to reduce the likelihood of "wrong site surgery," and the following comments parallel the AAOS recommendations:

1. In the holding area before the patient has been sedated, introduce yourself and chat with the patient for a minute. It will be easy to establish their identity as you compare their name and age with the chart.
2. Ask the patient to identify the limb undergoing surgery and to briefly describe the procedure he or she is about to undergo.
3. Mark the limb. Writing your initials on the limb is the AAOS suggestion. Make sure that your mark will remain visible after the patient is draped, so make the mark close to the area of the anticipated incision.
4. Corroborate this information with the side (right or left) noted in the chart history, the operative consent, the OR schedule, and the x-rays. (I also bring my office records to the OR as an additional method of confirmation.)
5. Check everything again as the patient is being prepped in the OR. You should see your mark on the limb and reconfirm that the proper side is being readied. Before making an incision, you should be able to see your mark nearby.

Although patient and side identity are ultimately the responsibility of the attending surgeon, it is never too early in surgical training to learn these important rituals.

X-RAYS

Some orthopaedic conditions do not require x-rays as part of the work-up, but most do. For those surgical conditions in which x-rays have been obtained, the films should be present in the OR when surgery is performed. Hanging the films should be part of your OR protocol. Furthermore, the films should be hung on a view box in an organized fashion and visible to the surgeon at all times. The *convention for hanging films* depends on whether the area in question is the spine or the extremities:

- For the spine, films are hung as if the surgeon is viewing the patient from behind, so the side marked "right" on the film is oriented on the right side of the viewbox.
- For everything else (extremities), the films are positioned as if the patient is standing facing you. For example, an x-ray of the right shoulder would be situated so that the shoulder is on the left side of the view box.

No matter how the films are positioned, make every attempt to have them situated so that the side marker (R or L) is visible. This is an additional way to help confirm the operative side. However, note that often both sides of any given patient will have been x-rayed, with films sitting in the film jacket.

For fracture cases, arthroscopy, joint replacement, tumor surgery, and anything else that involves bone work, the films should be sitting where you can see them. No pilot flies without a flight plan and map in the cockpit, and you shouldn't either.

STERILE TECHNIQUE

Orthopaedic surgeons may be the most neurotic of all surgical subspecialists with respect to sterile technique because infection so commonly spells catastrophe. Some patients undergoing total joint replacement who sustain a deep infection may never be able to undergo a successful arthroplasty procedure. For total joint replacement, many institutions use specialized equipment to reduce the likelihood of wound infection, such as ultraviolet lights (to kill airborne bacteria) or laminar airflow.

You should appreciate, then, the meticulous technique by which most orthopaedic patients are prepped and draped for surgery. Strict sterile technique is observed throughout the operation, and most staff wear two sets of gloves.

1. **Contamination:** Pay close attention to how you stand and what you touch. If you suspect you have broken sterile technique in any way, just tell the attending or scrub nurse. They will correct whatever potential contamination occurred. After a short time, you will gain your "sterile senses" and be able to function effortlessly without risking contamination.

2. **Double gloving:** A word about double gloving is warranted. If your gloves are too tight, your fingers will start to go numb after a just a few minutes. A simple adjustment helps greatly. Wear the inner layer as a half-size bigger than your normal size. For example, if your normal glove size is 7, first put on a half-size larger (7.5). Then, put on the outer gloves as a size 7. The slightly larger inner layer will not be too tight for your fingers, and the outer gloves will be snug enough that you won't lose tactile acuity.

SHARPS

Surgeons and OR staff are at risk for cutting themselves, because a large part of their time in the OR is spent around sharp instruments. Although most of these injuries might be viewed as minor inconveniences, they can in some cases become life threatening because of disease transmission from contaminated blood. Some statistics suggest that the transmission rate of human immunodeficiency virus (HIV) might be as high as 1 of 200 for a puncture wound caused by an instrument contaminated with infected blood. A less popularized, but perhaps much more likely threat, is the transmission of hepatitis. This disease can be not only severely debilitating, but also chronic and fatal.

As you can appreciate, the possibility of inadvertent needle sticks and lacerations is an occupational hazard that cannot be taken lightly. It is in your best interest (and of those around you) to learn preventive behavior:

1. Assume every patient you deal with may be HIV- or hepatitis-positive.
2. Wear gloves anytime you might touch blood or bodily fluids.
3. Once surgery is in progress, keep focused on the whereabouts of needles, knives, and any other cutting tools.
4. Hand instruments back to nurses or assistants by the handle first or with the needlepoint clamped into an instrument.
5. Do not make any sudden motions with sharp instruments or wave your hands about, even if your hands are empty. Many accidental punctures arise from the surgeon moving his or her hands *into* the sharp tool.
6. Do not struggle attempting to pass a heavy needle through tissue. If you cannot easily accomplish the maneuver in a controlled fashion, use two hands or get someone to help you. Sudden jerks will land the needle point-first in your other hand or in someone else's. This is particularly true when attempting to pass sharp steel trocars, as used in placing drains. These trocars are especially treacherous and require great attention on the part of everyone scrubbed so as to avoid accidental injury. Use two hands to place the trocar while someone else grabs the penetrating sharp end with a large clamp (like a Kocher).

Wearing two pairs of gloves will provide a small amount of extra protection against needle sticks. If you are struck or cut hard enough to draw your own blood, step out of the field, have the circulating nurse remove your gloves, assess the wound, and wash it with Betadine. Even if the injury is small, you should then contact the Infectious Disease Department at your institution (or Occupational Health) for further specific instructions on wound care and possible testing for disease transmission.

SPECIAL EQUIPMENT

Many orthopaedic procedures require tools or implants that must be ordered ahead of time specifically for the day of surgery. These items can range from a particular type of hip implant to a single special screw or drill bit. As a future orthopaedic attending physician, your ultimate responsibility one day will be to make the necessary arrangements that guarantee all equipment is on hand for the operation.

As a medical student or junior resident, it is unlikely that you will be directly involved with procuring special equipment for patients. However, with a little experience, you may be able to anticipate which operations will use special equipment. Try to talk with your attending or orthopaedic charge nurse, and get a copy of the protocol that describes the equipment. Technique tips are usually included in this literature, and you can be better prepared for the upcoming surgery.

PRACTICE MAKES PERFECT (ALMOST)

As you start to learn basic surgical skills, remember to practice as much as possible. Knot tying can be practiced almost anywhere, and even seemingly trivial tasks, such as using a suture scissors, have some subtlety and can be refined a great deal.

Many students and junior residents feel discouraged or intimidated at some point in their training because their skills seem to be substandard. Contrary to some opinion, however, very few surgeons are born with such good intrinsic motor skills that their professional development is effortless. In actuality, you will discover that the difference in skill level between one surgeon and another may be mostly a reflection of how many cases each physician has performed.

For example, a beginning knee arthroscopist may have performed only 50 cases and may still occasionally struggle with portal placement. In contrast, someone who has performed more than 500 knee arthroscopies usually appears smoother and more confident. Is the second surgeon a "born" arthroscopist, or is the difference really just about 450 cases more of experience?

There is no question that other factors play into the evolution of surgical talent, such as motor coordination and three-dimensional visualization, knowledge base, and organization. The latter two of these issues are discussed below. Just remember that practicing your skills and the accumulation of experience will have a tremendous impact on improving your technical abilities.

READING

It is crucial that you prepare for surgery by reading about the relevant pathology. If you read about a topic that you subsequently see directly—that is, by examining a patient or participating in the patient's surgery— you find it much easier to retain information indefinitely. Furthermore, most orthopaedic attending physicians appreciate the effort demonstrated by your attempt at preparing for cases. Check the OR schedule 1 or 2 days before each case, and invest some time in preparation. Some general reference sources are noted in Appendix F.

Anatomy is another topic that warrants your attention. You may note that some surgeons who seem to be confident and efficient are merely demonstrating excellent command of their anatomy knowledge base. The better you know the terrain, the faster and more safely you can proceed. A few helpful anatomy references are noted in Appendix F.

Remember, experience and motor skills are not enough to make a good orthopaedic surgeon. Book knowledge is another key piece of the pie.

PLANNING

Organizational skill may be the most underestimated feature of the good surgeon. Ironically, taking time to plan a case properly is easily under the surgeon's control and may have the greatest effect on the outcome of the operation.

Even though you may be a junior member of the surgical team, good planning is an excellent habit to develop early. Identify ahead of time the cases for which you will be scrubbing, and read about the patient's problem. Then, see if you can get a look at the x-rays and chart before the operation. If any implants or special hardware are to be used, read all you can about the equipment the day before surgery. Even as an attending physician, I still go through a specific ritual for every operation. Although much of the remaining discussion may not seem to be practically applicable to a medical student or junior resident, it will emphasize the importance of good planning and how seriously it is taken by attending physicians.

I make sure that the patient is reexamined in my office within 1 or 2 weeks before the day of surgery, just to make sure that nothing has changed in the history or physical exam. Special equipment needs are noted, and appropriate ordering is done, at the latest a week before surgery. An assessment is also made to make sure that any special studies (e.g., computed tomography scan, magnetic resonance imaging) are available.

Even if I know the patient well, the night before surgery I re-review my office records and carefully reevaluate the x-rays. Any special measurements are remeasured. Certain types of fracture patients require tracings or blueprint type drawings to facilitate efficient reconstruction of the fracture puzzle. When I was a resident, I wrote down concise notes outlining the key points (and any special equipment needs) for all the orthopaedic operations I attended. I kept a single notecard for each specific type of procedure. To this day I still review some of those notes; if I perform an unusual or new procedure, I create another card.

The process of writing out, or "storyboarding," an operation helps to organize the procedure in your mind and tends to iron out obstacles before they actually occur in surgery. Furthermore, you will recognize that most procedures can be divided into distinct parts: exposure, main procedure, and closure. Ideally, you should be able to plan how much time will be spent on each portion of the operation and thereby maximize your efficiency.

Remember that good organization decreases the likelihood of problems in the OR: "Chance favors the prepared mind." Wouldn't you rather fly with a pilot who had all the equipment checked, maps ready, routes planned, latest weather information, and time schedules already worked out? Or, what about the pilot who just got into the plane and took off, planning to "figure everything out as I go"?

If you are totally prepared, you will be able to operate faster without sacrificing safety. Operations tend to have easy parts and hard parts, all mixed together. Your goal is to go fast on the "straight-aways" and go slow on the "curves." The trick is to know what are the straight-aways and what are the curves. Good planning will help you tell the difference before you even put your gloves on.

15

CHAPTER

Special Equipment

This chapter provides an introduction to some of the specialized equipment commonly used in the orthopaedic operating room. An in-depth discussion of these instruments is beyond the scope of this text and requires further research on your part (see Appendix F for suggestions). Also, keep in mind that orthopaedic surgery is highly mechanical, and consequently some of the tools are complicated. Becoming comfortable with these procedures can take a long time (many operations or years of experience).

THE AO INSTRUMENTS

Operative management of broken bones often involves the placement of metal screws and plates. The design of the most commonly used fracture hardware system evolved from the work of a group of Swiss surgeons in the 1960s. The original name for the team of Swiss orthopaedists was the *Arbeitsgemein-schaft für Osteosynthesefragen*, and their system, which is still the gold standard for fracture care today, is referred to as the AO system. The design of the hardware and the tools to place it were based on certain key "AO" principles of fracture biology and the focus on achieving rigid internal fixation of the fracture.

A wide variety of AO equipment is now available in addition to the basic fracture trays, such as external fixators and fracture sets designed specifically for a

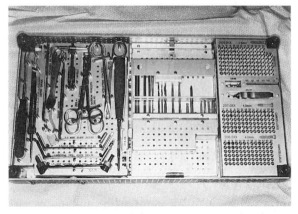

Figure 15–1. The AO small-fragment tray. Note that the necessary instruments (clamps, retractors, drill guides, and screwdrivers) are at the left. The center portion of the tray holds various drill bits and "taps." The right contains different types of screws in a variety of indicated lengths.

specific bone (e.g., distal radius, proximal femur). However, the basic fracture trays are still the cornerstones of most fracture care, because they contain most of the standard screws, plates, and most important, the tools to apply the hardware. The basic trays come in three sizes, based on the size of the bone in question:

1. The large-fragment set is generally used for the femur, tibia, and humerus.
2. The small-fragment set (Fig. 15–1) is helpful for intermediate-sized areas, such as the ankle, distal radius, and forearm bones.
3. The smallest set is the minifragment tray, which is usually limited to applications in the hand or the fixation of tiny articular fractures.

Note that, commonly, several trays are used on one fracture, because sometimes a mixture of screw sizes and instruments is necessary.

The AO fracture equipment has been specifically designed for application to bone. Almost every detail of the screw, plate, and tool design has been optimized to make each step of fracture surgery easier and increase the likelihood of healing:

1. For each diameter of screw, there is a matching drill
   bit that should be used to create the perfect pilot
   hole. A special guide is used to help hold the drill
   bit in proper position and prevent wrapping up soft
   tissue in the spinning bit.
2. A tool called a "depth gauge" is used to measure the
   appropriate length of screw needed.
3. A sharply threaded instrument called a "tap" is
   twisted into the pilot hole and cuts threads into the
   bone so that the screw does not create cracks at
   the hole.
4. The screw can then be placed, using a special hex-
   head screwdriver, which reduces the chances of slip-
   ping off the screw head.

Plates come in a wide range of sizes and shapes, all of
which are intended to address specific fracture patterns.
The contour of the plate, its thickness, and design of
its holes have all been carefully machined. For example,
certain plates called "dynamic compression" plates are
designed to have some of the screws placed slightly (0.1
to 0.5 mm) off axis from the center of the plate hole. A
customized drill guide allows reliable placement of the
bone hole (and subsequent screw placement) in this
slightly off center location. The hole in the plate is fash-
ioned with sloping sides, so that if an off-axis screw is
tightened down, it will slide the plate slightly (0.1 to
0.5 mm) in one direction. For certain fractures, this action is specifically used to create compression across
the fracture site, which can produce favorable fracture
mechanics and healing responses.

The AO equipment is highly technical, and its optimal
use requires significant practice and understanding.
Studying the AO principles allow you not only to better
master the precise techniques involved, but also to better understand the basic biology of fracture healing.

ARTHROPLASTY EQUIPMENT

Orthopaedic technology is constantly evolving, and
the design of major joint arthroplasty components
changes almost yearly. For example, the implants that
were used to perform hip and knee replacement during
my residency years have long vanished, having been

replaced by multiple design revisions over the past decade. A major trend in arthroplasty components has been not only improvement in the design of the implants themselves, but also improvement in the tools and guidance "jigs" that are used to place the components. A more traditional style of bone preparation involved making saw cuts by estimating with your eye and then just guessing. Modern instruments allow for much more precision. For example, special guides can be clamped onto the distal femur, and the necessary saw cuts for a total knee arthroplasty can then be made by resting the saw blade on a metal guide surface.

The best thing you can do to prepare for the technical aspects of arthroplasty cases is to obtain a current "protocol" brochure from the instrument sales representative. Study the protocol carefully, and pay particular attention to the correct sequence for use of the instruments.

ARTHROSCOPY EQUIPMENT

Arthroscopy can now be performed on almost every joint in the body, with the knee and shoulder being by far the most common sites. Arthroscopy requires a highly specialized operating room setup and equipment inventory. The main principle involves placement of a video telescope, usually about the diameter of a pencil (or smaller) into a joint distended with irrigation fluid. With the joint distended, it is then possible to inspect intracapsular anatomy with the telescope (the image is projected onto a television screen) and also place additional small tools into the joint for manipulation of tissue. The whole time this is being done, all instruments (including the arthroscope) enter the joint only through small, percutaneous incisions. If too large incisions were to be made, for example, fluid would leak out and joint distention would be lost.

Arthroscopy has become a science unto its own, allowing for completely new ways to treat certain types of pathology, and also accounting for better understanding of the joint pathology through better visualization.

There are two basic issues that you should understand about arthroscopy cases.

1. **The room and equipment setup must be performed with an eye for detail:** For example, arthroscopic inspection of the knee may appear to be relatively easy. However, the actual procedure occurs only after a long sequence of precise adjustments are made in how the patient's leg is positioned, how a special clamp holds the leg, where exactly the skin incisions are made for portal placement, as well as a whole host of other seemingly minor steps. It is the cumulative effect of all these minor details that allows the operation to proceed successfully. If any of these preparatory steps is omitted or executed poorly, what seems like a simple case can turn into a nightmarish struggle to accomplish even the most rudimentary surgical goal. Good arthroscopists have a mental checklist, which allows a systematic approach to setting up the room and all the equipment. Watch carefully how this "preparatory" phase occurs, from positioning the patient on the operating table to positioning the TV monitor. Proper setup is more than half the game.

2. **Technical skills are required to perform orthopaedic arthroscopy:** Although an experienced arthroscopist makes any given procedure look simple, the motor skills required are significantly different from those used in nonarthroscopic surgery. Arthroscopy requires the development of special hand-eye coordination, because the surgeon infrequently looks directly at the joint undergoing surgery. The surgeon is intensely focused on the TV monitor and not on his or her hands. Furthermore, the scope is held with one hand while the other hand usually holds an instrument, such as a probe or cutting tool. Therefore, both hands have to move independently while the information needed to adjust position and orientation is acquired by looking away from the surgical site at a video screen. With some experience, the surgeon is also able to help coordinate tools held in the left and right hands by sensing their relative location in space, a skill referred to as *triangulation.*

   The point you should remember is that acquisition of arthroscopy skills follows a learning curve that may be independent of whatever surgical skills you may already have. As in many other orthopaedic techniques, practice is the key.

FLUOROSCOPY

Certain operations necessitate the use of fluoroscopy. This is equivalent to a real-time, video x-ray. The fluoroscopy machine is often referred to as the "C-arm" because it has a giant C-shaped attachment that has an x-ray transmitter on one end and a receiver on the other end (Fig. 15–2). Anything placed in between the two will be imaged with x-rays and shown on a television-like monitor (attached by a cable to the C-arm). The C-arm itself is bulky, but with a few knob adjustments, is usually quite mobile so that it can be positioned almost anywhere.

Operations that require use of the C-arm are those in which an intraoperative "progress report" is necessary to ensure that the mechanical aspects of surgery are proceeding correctly. These operations typically include long-bone roddings, complex large-bone fracture cases, and many foot and hand surgery procedures. Use

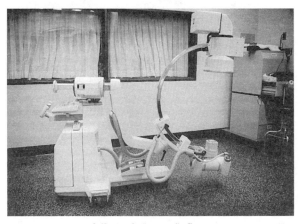

Figure 15–2. A full-sized "C-arm" fluoroscopy unit. Not shown is the (equally large) television monitor cabinet on which the x-ray images are displayed.

of fluoroscopy can save time because it is often used to quickly check the position of the first few screws or wires and to make sure that correct position is present or that a fracture is perfectly aligned. The key here is to check these issues *before* all the screws are placed and the hardware location has been committed. It is much easier to remove one screw and redrill a new hole than it is to remove 10 screws and a plate and start over. Furthermore, if all the screw holes have been drilled, starting over may be impossible because there may not be any more room for new holes.

Fluoroscopy units come in a variety of sizes and with a range of options. For example, small units ("mini-C-arms") are now available, which are specifically designed for foot and hand surgery and other small bone work (Fig. 15–3). These devices give off a smaller amount of radiation compared with the full-sized standard units, and their small size makes them more user-friendly in cramped quarters.

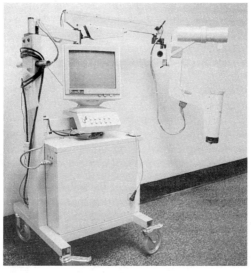

Figure 15–3. A "mini–C-arm" unit. Note that a compact display monitor is incorporated into the unit. These smaller fluoroscopes are convenient to use during hand and foot surgery.

Be aware of a few practical details with regard to the standard, full-sized fluoroscopy units:

1. Fluoroscopy units give off radiation, so everyone in the operating room should wear lead vests (and probably thyroid and eye protection) during their use. This includes the nurses, anesthesia staff, and the patient. One helpful role that you can assume is to procure the lead vests for everyone before the case starts. The vests are heavy and often dispersed throughout several operating suites. Don't forget to place a vest on the patient, covering the chest and pelvis (assuming that these areas are not in the field of surgery).

2. Positioning the equipment in the operating room can become time consuming, because many operating rooms are barely big enough to accommodate the staff, patient, and necessary orthopaedic instruments, let alone the imaging gear. Offer assistance to the radiology technician who operates the fluoroscopy machinery, because the C-arm and monitors are heavy and bulky. The radiology technician will be grateful for an extra set of helping hands in getting the room set up.

3. Learning how to move and connect the equipment yourself will constitute helpful skills when a "quick look" is needed in the middle of a case and the technician is temporarily tied up somewhere else.

16

Postoperative Documentation

Documentation after a surgical procedure constitutes a critical part of the medical record and is just as important as chart entries after emergency room care or inpatient rounds. The two principal tasks after surgery are the postoperative chart note and the operative record. Both should be created as soon as possible after the patient's surgery, preferably in the recovery room. As in any other medical care event, these notes represent the legal record of what actually happened in the operating room. Certain key elements for each of these entries are reviewed in this chapter.

THE POSTOPERATIVE NOTE

The postoperative note is typically written in the chart as the first entry after surgery. Make this entry the minute the patient is secure in the recovery room. Some hospitals actually have a stamp that allows you to imprint a page in the chart and then just fill in the blanks. The following list is an example of a standard, complete postoperative note.

1. Preoperative diagnosis
2. Postoperative diagnosis
3. Procedure
4. Surgeon
5. Assistant(s)

6. Anesthesia modality
7. Estimated blood loss
8. Fluids administered during surgery: _____ mL crystalloid, _____ mL blood
9. Urine output
10. Tourniquet time
11. Drains
12. Specimens sent to pathology
13. Cultures sent to microbiology
14. Operative findings
15. Implants
15. Patient status in recovery room

Although making entries in the list may seem like a lot of writing, you need to get in the habit of entering a complete note after every case. Although many elements of this note will be repeated in the dictated operative record, the actual operative record may not be transcribed or placed in the chart for several days. The postoperative note, then, is the only tangible record of surgery that is available in the chart.

Do not underestimate the value of documenting the fluid balance maintained during surgery. These details can become critically important. For example, if the patient becomes unstable after surgery, the medical resuscitation team may need to know how much fluid was administered. Also state whether the patient received blood.

In fact, orthopaedic patients as a group will predictably experience a variety of problems postoperatively, related not only to the patient's preexisting medical status, but also to anesthetic administration, blood loss, tourniquet ischemia, and orthopaedic implant placement. A few examples of medical situations that require acute therapy include pulmonary edema, heart failure due to fluid overload, pulmonary embolus, myocardial infarction, hip dislocation after arthroplasty, and peroneal nerve palsy after knee arthroplasty. The details of the operative note allow intelligent intervention to proceed in managing any of these problems.

DICTATING THE PROCEDURE

The operative note is one of the most important written entries in the medical record. It functions as the absolute record of what happened during surgery. In any situation in which the events or outcome of surgery are contested, the operative note will be dissected and analyzed word for word. Although dictating the operative note is usually regarded as a chore to be foisted on the least senior resident available, it takes some skill to create a good operative summary.

General Principles

The following are important principles in creating the operative note:

1. **If you weren't present during the procedure (or do not understand what was done), do not dictate the record:** This is perhaps the most fundamental principle in creating the operative note. Sounds ridiculously obvious, doesn't it? It's not. Somebody may casually remark to you at the end of a case, "Oh, be a good chap and dictate the case for me." Sometimes, you may have been present only during the closure or, conversely, during the main part of the procedure but not during the closure. Or you may have just seen that particular operation for the first time and still are not sure how everything was done. If you are not certain that you can dictate a logical and highly accurate account of everything that took place during surgery, do not dictate the report. Tell your superior—whether a resident or even the attending physician—that you didn't see everything or that you need to see another case before you dictate a good note. You cannot afford to dictate what you "assumed" took place, nor should the report be vague or imprecise.

2. **Dictate the record as soon as possible after surgery:** The ideal time is as soon as the patient arrives in the recovery room. The operation will be fresh in your head and it will be the easiest to dictate an accurate summary. If you have to postpone the dictation for some reason, do not let more than 24 hours pass from the time of surgery without dictating. You will be amazed at how much harder it is to record all the details easily if you wait more than a day.

3. **Be objective:** You should not use language that is emotional, inflammatory, or mysterious. Be as de-

scriptive as possible, but do not attempt to "argue" some point of view, place blame, or be derogatory about the patient, anesthesia staff, or anyone else. For example, if a large blood loss occurred, mention the bleeding in the dictation. However, do not state, "we couldn't control the bleeding." Not only does that sound bad for the surgeon, it typically isn't true. Excessive blood loss is commonly caused by anticoagulation medication, coagulopathy, reaming a long bone, or even patient obesity. Of course, also don't state, "the patient was so fat that he bled a lot." It's better to say that bleeding was encountered (state about how much and where) and that it was controlled (state how). Words like "inadvertently" or "accidentally" suggest a degree of sloppiness or inattentiveness that are also suboptimal for an operative note. Try to use objective language and stick to describing the facts of surgery dispassionately.

Standard Elements

Your operative notes will benefit from being organized and complete. Listed below are certain "standard" items that routinely belong in the note:

1. **Demographics of the dictation:** State *your name* (and spell it) as the dictating party and then state, and spell the *patient's name.* List the patient's *social security* or medical record number, and then the *date of the operation.* Also note the *location of the procedure* (hospital or center name).

2. **Procedure title:** This requires noting a *preoperative diagnosis, postoperative diagnosis,* and *procedure.* Note here also the *method of anesthesia.* Then list the name of the *principal surgeon,* and list any *assistants,* in order of involvement.

3. **Introduction:** Many surgeons prefer to include an introduction, although it is not always necessary. Here, a brief history of the patient's problem and treatment course is described, creating a logical course that ends with the decision to proceed with surgery. This "introductory" segment is often used to clearly demonstrate the indications for surgery. Often, mention is made that the patient underwent

informed consent and was also instructed as to the potential risks of surgery as well as treatment alternatives.

4. **Main body of the dictation:** Begin dictating the formal procedure. It is helpful to restate where the procedure was performed, what anesthetic was administered, in what position on the table the patient was placed, and that the patient's identity and the correct extremity were identified. Then, dictate the procedure as it occurred chronologically. If more than one operation was performed or if bone graft was obtained, include details as to how this was done.

5. **Conclusion:** At the end of the operative note, dictate a final paragraph that addresses the patient's exit from the operating room. If general anesthesia was used, note that the patient was awakened and extubated. It is a good idea to document that the sponge, needle, and instrument counts were reported as correct. If a tourniquet was used, note the tourniquet time. Describe the dressing applied, and indicate that the patient was safely transported back to the recovery room or holding area. As a final note, if you or the surgeon speaks with the patient and family postoperatively, it is a good idea to document that fact. I usually dictate that I spoke with the patient (and family members, if present) about the operative details, and that follow-up instructions were explained and provided in writing.

A Sample Operative Note

It might be helpful to review an actual operative note in its entirety. What follows is one of my standard dictations for an endoscopic carpal tunnel release.

This is Leon S. Benson, B-E-N-S-O-N, dictating an operative note on Jane Doe, D-O-E, medical record number 123-45-6789. Date of surgery was 1/10/99 at Evanston Hospital. Preoperative diagnosis was right carpal tunnel syndrome; postoperative diagnosis, same. Procedure was right endoscopic carpal tunnel release. Surgeon was Dr. Benson, first assistant was Dr. John Resident. Anesthesia method was Bier block.

Procedure: The patient was identified and taken to the operating room at Evanston Hospital on 1/10/99, placed supine on the operating table where she underwent administration of a right-upper-extremity Bier block by the Division of Anesthesia. The patient then had a sterile prep and drape of the right upper extremity in the usual fashion, and all bony prominences were carefully padded during positioning of the patient and extremity.

Next, landmarks were marked on the skin with a marking pen in the usual fashion for endoscopic approach to the carpal tunnel. The proximal portal was made first by making a transverse incision between the proximal and distal wrist flexion creases and between the flexor carpi ulnaris and palmaris longus tendons. Subcutaneous fat was bluntly dissected and superficial veins were electrocauterized. The underlying antebrachial fascia was then clearly identified and cut with a No.15 blade in such a way as to create a rectangular-shaped, distally based flap. This flap was then elevated distally, and it was then possible to introduce a curved elevator beneath it. The undersurface of the transverse carpal ligament was then easily palpable, and the typical washboard effect of its transverse fibers was easily appreciated. The elevator was then used to palpate the distal margin of the transverse carpal ligament, and this margin correlated nicely with the marking in the palm denoting the distal portal.

The distal portal was then made by making a longitudinal, 5-mm-long incision in line with the ring finger ray overlying the distal margin of the transverse carpal ligament. Subcutaneous fat and fascia were then bluntly dissected through the distal portal under direct vision. It was then possible to introduce the endoscopic cannula and obturator assembly through the proximal portal, underneath the transverse carpal ligament, and out through the distal portal. The obturator was then removed and the hand was placed in slight extension in the hand holder. It was now possible to introduce the arthroscope and instruments from either end of the cannula.

Arthroscopic inspection demonstrated clearly the transverse, white fibers of the transverse carpal ligament. No intervening neurovascular or tendinous structures were noted. The ligament was palpated with a probe and its appearance correlated with its palpation. The central portion of the ligament was then incised longitudinally with a triangle knife, and this cut was then continued proximally and distally using the hook knife. The central portion of the ligament was quite thick. Consequently, several cuts with the triangle knife were necessary to completely release the ligament. However, once these cuts were accomplished, the ligament completely separated by at least 5 mm, and fat herniated from above the ligament down between the cut edges, verifying a complete release. The released area was also reprobed, and no remaining fibers were palpated. It was also easy to rotate the cannula from side to side and inspect the cut edges of each side of the ligament, again confirming that the ligament was completely released. Final inspection again demonstrated no intervening neurovascular or tendinous structures.

Next, the obturator was replaced into the cannula, and the obturator-cannula assembly was removed intact from the hand. The portals were copiously irrigated, and then the skin wounds were closed with simple stitches of 5-0 nylon sutures. A Bacitracin and Adaptic dressing was then applied to both wounds, and then the hand was incorporated into a bulky forearm based dressing incorporating a forearm based volar plaster splint.

Once the dressing was secure, the tourniquets for the Bier block were released, tourniquet time being 32 minutes. Excellent vascularity returned to the tips of all fingers when the tourniquet was released. The patient was then moved on a cart from the operating room to recovery in excellent condition. All sponge, needle, and instrument counts were reported as correct. After the patient was in recovery, the details of surgery were reviewed with the patient and the family in the family waiting area. All of their questions were answered, and detailed care and follow-up instructions were explained and provided in writing.

This concludes the operative note for Jane Doe, D-O-E, dictated by Leon S. Benson, M.D. Thank you.

4
PART

Clinic and Conference

17
CHAPTER

The Orthopaedic Office

The orthopaedic office deserves special mention because, on a weekly basis, you may spend more than 10% or 20% of your time there. Although many training programs traditionally have stressed emergency room (ER) and operating room experiences, the "clinic" environment is another key element in learning orthopaedic care.

GO TO THE OFFICE

The first and simplest rule is to show up. Unfortunately, many students and residents believe that the office is a waste of time. They believe that the operating room must always be the priority, followed by the ER. Office hours are reserved only for situations when "there's nothing better to do," and these situations are to be avoided if at all possible.

The smart house officer knows that exposure to office orthopaedics is invaluable. Just as operating skills are essential to becoming a surgeon, office savvy will define you as a physician. You need to be able to distinguish surgical from nonsurgical pathology, and you need to know how to manage the nonsurgical problems, which tend to vastly outnumber those "interesting" surgical cases. Remember that your image as a competent surgeon may hinge less upon how well you can perform an operation and more on how you counsel your patients in the office.

When you are an attending, many more patients may rave about your injection skills and bedside manner than about your actual surgical proficiency. The converse may be true as well. For example, misreading a simple diagnosis, such as a trigger finger (flexor tendinitis), may cause the patient to complain bitterly that "Dr. Doe just doesn't seem to know how to help me." Although this may not seem proper or fair, the fact is that in the course of a week, you will probably have 10 to 20 times more patient encounters in the office than you will have operations. Moreover, each of your patients' problems—no matter how insignificant or uninteresting they may appear to you—is important to the patient.

Learn how to focus on each patient so that he or she feels that the problem is being appropriately addressed. After all, the patient is paying for this time to get a professional opinion. How you behave in front of the office audience will do more to create your orthopaedic persona than almost anything else.

Learning office skills requires time and patience. Plan to spend at least half a day every week with an attending physician seeing patients. Two half-days per week would be better. It can take years to feel comfortable dealing with the myriad situations that arise in the office setting, and you should not skimp on your office orthopaedic training.

YOUR ROLE: PASSIVE VERSUS ACTIVE

Many students feel that they are not doing a good job if they do not actively "do" something when patients are being seen. Although this is not a bad trait, performing procedures should not be the main focus of your office time. You are not there to make sure that the office runs smoothly. The following are suggestions on how to fulfill your role in the orthopaedic office:

1. Spend time observing the interaction between the attending physician and his or her patients. Pay attention to how the attending physician talks to pa-

tients and how much time is spent on explaining orthopaedic pathology in terms that a layperson can understand. The orthopaedic office is typically a very busy place.

2. Try to learn how all the ancillary staff function together, including nurses, secretaries, schedulers, receptionists, and technical staff. Do not hesitate to simply follow the attending physician and observe numerous patient encounters. Because every attending physician may be slightly different, a good idea would be to first discuss your role within the office so that both of you can be clear on your duties. Remember that although taking a history, performing the physical exam, applying casts, and giving injections may eventually become part of your experience, there is always someone to perform these tasks if you are not there. Your main goals should be to learn basic office orthopaedic care and become familiar with the typical rhythm of the office setting.

3. Carry a note card or small paper pad and write down particular diagnoses or even just terminology that you hear in the office. Taking notes such as these can be very helpful. You can later look up specific conditions or observations so that you will learn more details about what you saw or heard. As you probably already know, you will remember a condition or physical finding far longer if you personally observed or examined a patient with that problem. So make a list during each office experience, and then spend 5 minutes reading about each item before the next office day. You will be amazed at how much you learn and retain.

MAIN TYPES OF OFFICE PATIENTS

It may be helpful to categorize office visits into four main categories:

1. **The new patient:** This patient usually requires the most time, because an introductory history and physical exam are required. Furthermore, identification of pathology and explanation of the condition in addition to treatment options may consume a fair amount of time and effort.

2. **The ER follow-up patient:** This patient is very similar to the new patient, except that the condition in question is usually related to trauma (e.g., fracture, laceration). ER follow-up patients may also require a fair amount of time, depending on the seriousness of their injuries and whether further care is required. Cast applications and dressing changes are often necessary, and a few of these patients may require additional intervention such as surgery. ER follow-up patients, therefore, can be unpredictably labor intensive. Some may require nothing more than suture removal or a bandage, whereas others may require a lengthy review of alternative treatments, casting, or a preoperative discussion.
3. **The established patient:** This patient has been seen before and is following up for continuing care. These visits tend to be more focused because the problem has usually already been identified and a full history and physical exam are not necessary. Any change in symptoms or physical exam findings are often carefully noted.
4. **The postoperative patient:** Visits with these patients are often quick and easy (assuming no complications have occurred). Dressing changes, suture removal, and a review of ongoing physical or occupational therapy make up the main activities.

Categorizing patients into these four groups may help you understand what the patient will expect (and need) from you in the office interaction. Furthermore, you may notice that mixing different types of visits on the same day tends to reduce the likelihood that the office schedule runs late, because the few patients that require more time may be offset by the interspersing of simpler, quicker visits.

Even though one can generally predict how complicated an office visit may be based on the categories just discussed, a seemingly simple visit may require a great deal of time if the patient is anxious or dissatisfied with his or her progress or care. No matter what type of patient you see, be sensitive enough to give each person the time and attention needed. You will notice that most attending physicians will not sacrifice the quality of their time with a patient just because the office is behind schedule.

18
CHAPTER

Fracture Conference

Fracture conference is the prototypical orthopaedic presentation environment, in which students and residents are expected to present cases in front of an audience. This brief chapter highlights a few principles that might make your morning at the podium a little easier. Although the main reference here is the hypothetical "fracture" conference, you will eventually be exposed to other types of academic settings for which the following principles also apply (i.e., tumor conference, morbidity and mortality conference).

PREPARATION

Reading

Before the conference begins, you must be ready. Preparation is the key ingredient to looking good. In fact, you must *overprepare*, if possible, to compensate for the fact that your audience (typically attendings and senior residents) will know more than you.

1. First, *learn about the topic*. Make use of what few natural advantages you have in the conference scenario when you are the presenter: You know what the case is, and you have this information ahead of time. Therefore, read as much as you can to arm yourself with facts.

2. Even if you think you know enough about the particular case to discuss it intelligently, *read a little more.* The more you know, the better you will be able to answer questions from the audience and discuss nuances of treatment and outcome.

3. *Focus on postoperative rehabilitation and outcomes.* A favorite line of questioning that often befuddles the junior houseofficer relates to posttreatment care. In fracture discussion, many presenters make the mistake of reading only about how to operate on a particular injury or how to classify the radiographic findings. You must also know about postoperative care and practical issues, which attending physicians love to ask. For example, an attending physician may ask these types of questions:

   "How soon will your ankle fracture patient be able to put full weight on her leg?"
   "Is physical therapy necessary?"
   "When can sports be resumed?"
   "Do you tell her that her ankle motion will ever be normal?"
   "When will it be normal?"

   Even if you cannot find exact answers the night before while you're reading, just giving these issues a little thought on your own will go a long way in reducing your anxiety when they "pop up" during the conference.

   Sources that are helpful to read come in two varieties.

1. The first and most basic source is the "standard" textbook. Examples include Rockwood and Green's fracture text or the orthopaedic trauma textbook by Chapman and associates. One of the best "standard-of-care"–type references is the *Orthopaedic Knowledge Update,* published by the American Academy of Orthopaedic Surgeons (see Appendix F). This material is critically written, very concise and to the point, and is updated every 3 years. Furthermore, there are individual volumes that deal with specialty subjects, including one just on trauma.

2. Another great source of information comes from *The Journal of the American Academy of Orthopaedic Surgeons: A Comprehensive Review.* These articles are tightly written, contemporary review papers that

deal with individual topics. This journal and the *Orthopaedic Knowledge Update* are an absolute must.

Other good information comes from current, specific journal articles and review papers. This material can be absorbed if you have the luxury of additional time, and they will increase the depth of your knowledge.

X-rays

Although your oral discussion of any given topic is important, the main act of almost any orthopaedic conference consists of the x-rays. You must have good x-rays to show for your case. The following are important suggestions for your preparation of x-rays:

1. The films you show should be able to tell the whole story by themselves. That is, you need (1) injury films, (2) postreduction films, (3) preoperative films, and (4) postoperative films. Do not panic if any given set of x-rays is of poor quality; just state that these were the x-rays obtained.

2. If you find yourself with a large collection of x-rays the night before the conference, go through them carefully and select the best studies. The ideal situation is to have just the right amount of x-rays to show. If you do not have postoperative x-rays, the audience will be irritated. No matter how many times you say that the operation went great and the reduction was perfect, the audience wants to draw its own conclusions. If you do not have enough films to radiographically document a case, it is probably better not to present the case at all. Too many films can also be a liability. You will frustrate the audience if you show a million different x-rays, most of which don't add anything to the presentation. Select the relevant x-rays and keep your radiographic data concise.

3. Sort the x-rays in advance. A classic mistake is to attempt to sort the films during the conference. It is considered poor form to sit in the back row awaiting your turn at the podium while furiously sorting through a heavy film jacket. It not only demonstrates poor preparation, but it is also rude because flipping films creates enough noise to distract attention from

the ongoing case. Even worse is when the presenter attempts to sort films while actually presenting the case. Invariably, films scatter onto the floor, or that critical postoperative view just can't be found when you desperately need it. Don't let this be you.
4. Look at all your films on a lightbox the night before the conference. Pick the ones you want to show and arrange them in the correct order. You can even use a crayon or china marker to number the films so that if they are dropped, you can still immediately show them in the right sequence. Writing the number in a specific location on every film, such as the top right, also helps with orienting the films on the lightbox. It can be embarrassing to hang an x-ray and start discussing your case when someone in the audience gently points out that the film is upside down.

PRESENTATION TECHNIQUE

The fracture conference is certainly not run the same way at every institution, so pay attention to how the cases are traditionally presented at your particular program. However, certain general principles hold true for most orthopaedic case presentations:

1. Provide concise information that allows the case details to be quickly appreciated by the audience. Your role is that of an information provider.
2. Be prepared to conduct some discussion that highlights key features of diagnosis and treatment. A simple organization method for your presentation is as follows:
   a. Patient history, physical exam, and possible mechanism of injury
   b. Radiographic findings
   c. Fracture classification
   d. Treatment alternatives
      1) Nonoperative
      2) Operative
   e. Rehabilitation issues
   f. Complications
3. Be prepared to stop anywhere in the discussion to allow more detailed discussion of any particular

point. In other words, having a discussion plan is great, but do not be so committed to it that you quash any interesting commentary that arises during your presentation. Remember that in addition to reviewing basic principles of care, this conference should also help elicit constructive academic discussion. Allowing some of this discussion to develop spontaneously is good.

4. Stand so that you do not block the audience's view of the x-rays.

MENTAL TOUGHNESS

The concept here is simple: *Do not be embarrassed if you are wrong.* In fact, expect to be wrong every time you present a case. Your audience knows more than you even if you read every book in the library the night before conference. Many residents and students strongly believe that a "good" presentation involves knowing the answer to every question posed by the audience, and a "bad" presentation is characterized by not knowing all the answers.

Unfortunately, nothing could be further from the truth. A good presentation is well organized and demonstrates some preparation on the part of the presenter. The presenter is calm, speaks clearly and deliberately, has all the films ready to go, and has an outline of what is important to discuss for the case at hand. Although you may feel vulnerable or uncomfortable after giving a wrong answer, the fact is that in the presentation of a well-organized, smartly presented case, most wrong answers are generally forgotten by the attending physicians as soon as conference is over. The lasting impression you make on your superiors will be through your style and poise, not by the numbers of points scored with correct guesses.

Conferences are not game shows, and good intention and underlying intelligence count a lot, even if your actual answer misses the mark occasionally. If you don't know the answer to a question, say so. Then take your best guess. Whether you're right or wrong, pay attention to the discussion, note the right answer, and move on. Nobody will think less of you.

19
CHAPTER

Differential Diagnosis in the Conference Setting

This last chapter deals with a common issue that strikes fear in the heart of the trainee—the "unknown case." An attending physician may bring a case and ask you as the student to figure it out. A one-sentence history is given, films are displayed on a view box, and someone points to you and says, "Hey, what's this?"

The reason why this situation deserves special mention is that most students and residents play the game the wrong way. It is tremendously tempting to look at the films and take a wild guess. Then if you're wrong, you take another guess, and so on, until you run out of guesses and feel like an idiot. If you have been manipulated into taking wild shots at your target, the odds are you'll never hit it. Furthermore, you will demonstrate very little knowledge in the process, so your answer will represent the sum total of what you know (and your answer is often wrong).

THE LIST: HOW TO ORGANIZE YOUR ANSWER

Actually, there's a simple solution to the problem of differential diagnosis. Instead of starting out with a single, definitive guess, start out very broadly and then meticulously narrow down your choices one by one. This way, even if you draw the wrong final conclusion, chances are most of your discussion will have had logical and academic value.

For any orthopaedic problem, there are about eight main categories that might describe the problem. Although the following list is not the only way to organize pathology (or necessarily the most complete list), it works well for most situations:

1. Trauma
2. Infection
3. Metabolic disorder
4. Tumor
5. Circulatory disorder
6. Synovial condition
7. Congenital or developmental condition
8. Degenerative disease

Learn this list (or a similar one) and try to see whether the case might fit into any of these categories first. How do you do this? You need to ask the appropriate "screening" questions.

BECOME THE QUESTIONER

It is helpful to follow these guidelines when dealing with the "unknown case":

1. **Start by taking the history:** Your questions should follow the same plan as if you were working up a patient in the emergency room (ER) or on the inpatient floor. Past medical problems, previous surgery, allergies, medications, family history, and review of systems are all appropriate issues to pursue.
2. **Ask your questioner for details of the physical exam:** Be sure to ask about areas of swelling, discoloration, tenderness, crepitus, and deformity; document range of motion, strength, and neurovascular function. Don't forget vital signs, especially temperature.
3. **Proceed to ask for x-rays and imaging studies, if necessary:** X-rays will probably be shown to you, but insist on getting the correct views. Remember

that for fractures, the films should show one joint above and below the injury area. At least two orthogonal films should be available. Look for both bone and soft-tissue detail on the films. If necessary, ask for additional imaging such as magnetic resonance imaging, computed tomography scan, or bone scan. The worst thing that can happen is that your questioner will deny access to the requested study. So, if it makes some sense to do so, ask for extra data.

4. **Consider ordering lab tests:** A complete blood count, sedimentation rate, blood chemistries, hormone levels, and tuberculin skin test are good examples. What you should be doing is verbally "working up" the patient.

5. **Return to your magic pathology list of eight items:** Your attempt to deduce the correct diagnosis should result from the overlap of the patient's history, physical exam, and objective testing. Once you have drawn this information from your examiner, orally run through your list. In fact, start by stating the following: *Based on the history, physical exam, and objective tests so far available, the following conclusions can be drawn.* Then, run through your list aloud, item by item, including the categories that seem possibly correct and excluding the categories that do not fit with the data.

SAMPLE CASE

You are given a case in which a 66-year-old man presents with knee pain. Films are hung up that show erosive changes about the tibia and femur. Should you just guess that it must be arthritis? No. You will probably be wrong, if only because arthritis is such an obvious possibility that few attending physicians would show such a case in conference.

First, ask about the history and physical exam. Is the patient an African-American? Could this be sickle cell disease? (Yes) How long has the problem been present? Any history of trauma? Does the patient have a fever? After the physical exam, get lab studies. Is there a high white count? Has the knee been tapped? If it has, what are the synovial fluid chemistries? Is the patient malnourished? (Cancer) Any other lesions in the skeleton elsewhere? (Bone scan?)

Once you've obtained information, go through your list as follows:

> Based on the history, physical exam, and objective tests so far available, the following conclusions can be drawn. Trauma is a possibility because this patient may have a stress fracture through a preexisting defect, although the films do not show this clearly. So, I would place trauma (fracture) as a possibility, but an unlikely one. Infection is a definite consideration because some infections (e.g., tuberculosis) can cause x-ray changes similar to these and because the patient has some findings consistent with a slow, progressive infection (low-grade fever, progressive pain, chronic swelling). A metabolic condition is unlikely because the patient's lab tests are normal and the x-ray findings are not consistent with common endocrinologic disorders. The process could be a tumor, but it would have to be one that affects both sides of the joint and, therefore, advanced or represented by multiple metastases (unlikely). A circulatory condition is possible, specifically chronic sickle cell disease, given the radiographic findings, clinical course, and positive sickle cell test. A synovial condition is also possible because both sides of the joint line are affected, although with normal lab results this diagnosis might depend on a synovial biopsy. A congenital condition is not supported by any of the data. Degenerative pathology such as osteoarthritis is highly possible, although low-grade fever and changes limited to just one joint make this diagnosis slightly suspect.
>
> To summarize, I would include infection, circulatory pathology, and degenerative disease as the three main possibilities. I think infection is the best guess, given the information presented. Furthermore, if I had to be specific, I would guess tuberculosis as a possible answer, although joint cultures and synovial biopsy data would be helpful.

After you say all that, does it really matter if you're right? Chances are you *will* be right or at least partially right. But even if the diagnosis turns out to be sickle cell disease or some strange form of arthritis, you will still appear knowledgeable. Why? Because you weren't just guessing. You went through a methodical process of working up the patient based on those old reliable processes: history, physical exam, and objective testing. And then you went through your master list and discussed each item, including or excluding it based on merits of the case in question. You started from a broad base and systematically narrowed down the possibilities until you were left with only a few logical choices. Answering an unknown problem such as this with an audience will take some practice, because a fair amount of poise is required to "spar" with your examiner. However, you can learn the list (or create your own) and start to attack the problem properly. No one is impressed with wild guesses; if you're right, most people will think it was an accident.

Appendixes

A

APPENDIX

Overview of Multiple-Trauma Management

This appendix briefly reviews the assessment of patients with multiple trauma. Although an attending surgeon from the general surgery service will usually be the "team leader" for these patients, orthopaedic surgeons are often directly involved, and it is, therefore, helpful to be familiar with initial assessment concepts.

The following comments for trauma assessment are derived from the Advanced Trauma Life Support System, developed by the Committee on Trauma of the American College of Surgeons in an effort to improve the emergency care of patients with multiple trauma. The overall plan involves progression through four key stages of care: (1) primary survey, (2) resuscitation, (3) secondary survey, and (4) definitive care.

PRIMARY SURVEY

When the patient first arrives in the emergency room, you should attempt to obtain a brief history from the patient or other personnel (transport staff, witnesses, etc.). Then begin the primary survey. The goal here is to detect life-threatening problems and treat them as they are identified. The primary survey is organized according to the "ABCs." More specifically, the mnemonic is "ABCDE," which stands for *A*irway, *B*reathing, *C*irculation, *D*isability, and *E*xpose.

Airway means inspecting and clearing the airway of any obstructions, such as blood, loose teeth, foreign objects, or vomit. The cervical spine must always be protected during this stage because you *cannot* assume that the spine is stable. The presence of any head or facial trauma should make you even more suspicious of cervical spine pathology.

If the patient is unconscious or not breathing, you must clear the airway. First, the airway can be swept manually to clear it; if this doesn't work, a chin lift or manual jaw thrust may help. If the airway is now clear, an oral or nasopharyngeal airway device can be placed to maintain a clear path. If the airway cannot be cleared or maintained, then intubation is the next step. Remember, throughout this whole process, the cervical spine must be controlled carefully. Intubation is indicated specifically in patients with:

- An unstable or insecure airway
- Inadequate or labored breathing (patient gray, cyanotic, respiratory rate >35/minute)
- Lack of consciousness (especially with a closed-head injury)
- Deteriorating blood oxygenation
- Specific injuries that compromise the cardiopulmonary axis (flail chest, severe shock, pulmonary contusion, inhalation or facial burns, etc.)

If intubation is impossible (foreign object obstruction or severe maxillofacial trauma), then a cricothyroidotomy may be required to save the patient's life.

Breathing means that you must ensure that the patient has adequate ventilation through the airway you just secured. First, inspect the chest for flail segments, open wounds, or deformity. Palpate for tenderness or crepitus, which would suggest rib fractures. Then auscultate for the presence and quality of breath sounds bilaterally. Decreased breath sounds may indicate a pneumothorax, hemothorax, tension pneumothorax or hemothorax, or diaphragmatic rupture. If a tension pneumothorax or hemothorax is present, a large-bore needle or chest tube will improve the patient's physiology.

Pericardial tamponade is another life-threatening condition that may be identified by "Beck's triad" of presenting conditions:

- Elevated central venous pressure (distended neck veins)
- Decreased arterial pressure (narrowed pulse pressure)
- Muffled heart sounds

Treatment requires pericardiocentesis (placement of a needle into the pericardium); return of unclotted blood is both diagnostic and therapeutic for this condition.

Circulation assessment is the third phase of the primary survey. This requires evaluation of blood volume and peripheral perfusion. *Shock* is defined as a circulatory abnormality in which end-organ oxygenation is compromised through inadequate perfusion. Methods of assessment include palpating for pulses:

- A radial pulse suggests a systolic blood pressure of 80 or greater.
- A femoral pulse suggests a blood pressure of 70 or greater.
- A palpable carotid pulse suggests a pressure of 60 or greater.

Pulse rate, skin color and temperature, and capillary refill (<2 seconds is normal) are also examination points that help in evaluating blood volume. Remember that direct measurement of blood pressure alone may be a poor indicator of shock; 25% of blood volume can be lost without causing acute hypotension.

The fourth part of the primary survey is *disability* assessment. This involves a quick review of the patient's neurologic status and evaluation of the extremities for serious injury. The Glasgow Coma Scale is useful to rate basic neurologic function (Table A–1). Examination of the extremities should include assessment of motor and sensory function and distal blood flow. All long bones and extremity joints should be quickly palpated to identify potential fractures.

The last element of the primary survey is *expose.* This is a reminder to completely disrobe the patient so that no serious injuries are missed. Although this admonishment may seem unnecessary, it actually can be quite easy to miss a back or pelvic injury because the patient

Table A–1. GLASGOW COMA SCALE

Eye Opening	
Spontaneous	4 points
To voice	3
To pain	2
None	1
Verbal Response	
Oriented	5
Confused	4
Inappropriate words	3
Incomprehensible sounds	2
None	1
Motor Response	
Obeys commands	6
Purposeful movement	5
Withdraws to pain	4
Flexion to pain	3
Extension to pain	2
None	1
Total Score = 3–15	

is clothed and lying on a backboard. It must be standard protocol to remove clothing and inspect the entire body. The patient may be safely log-rolled to one side (protect the cervical spine) so that the back of the body can be inspected. Now is also the time to make sure that appropriate pelvic and rectal exams are performed. The morbidity of a missed rectal tear (caused by a pelvic fracture) is huge.

RESUSCITATION

As the primary survey proceeds, resuscitation should be conducted almost simultaneously. As noted above, if the airway is obstructed or unstable, clearing and securing it (intubation if necessary) are performed immediately. Often supplemental oxygen is provided here. During the "breathing" assessment, chest tubes may be placed, or needle decompression of tension pneumothorax or hemothorax may be indicated. Pericardial tamponade should be immediately decompressed. The circulation assessment will identify the patient's volume status. This phase of the primary survey is accompanied by placement of two large-bore (14-gauge) IV lines to facilitate rapid volume resuscitation. Two to three liters of warm crystalloid fluid is usually used for immediate volume replenishment. A general rule is to replace 3 milliliters of crystalloid for every milliliter of estimated blood loss. Basic monitoring should be repeated frequently to assess the patient's response to resuscitation; this includes checking vital signs, central neurologic function (mental status, etc.), pulse oximetry, urine output, and ECG patterns. The most important lab test is a type and crossmatch for packed red cells. Additional helpful tests include blood gases, complete blood count, electrolyte levels, amylase level, coagulation profile, and a toxic substance screen and alcohol level.

SECONDARY SURVEY

The point of the primary survey and resuscitation phase is to keep the patient from immediately dying from an obvious (and usually correctable) condition. Once the patient has been at least temporarily stabilized, you may begin the secondary survey. Remember that the primary survey and concomitant initial resuscitation should be completed within the first few minutes after the patient's arrival in the emergency room.

The secondary survey consists of a more complete history and physical exam. The body can be divided into specific regions that should be thoroughly examined: head and neck, chest, abdomen, genitourinary, and extremities. During the secondary survey, radiographic assessment is completed. The minimum trauma series includes a set of cervical spine films (lateral, anteroposterior, open-mouth view), an anteroposterior pelvic film, and an anteroposterior chest x-ray. Wounds are dressed with sterile bandages, fractures are splinted appropriately, antibiotics are started, and tetanus prophylaxis is administered. Nasogastric tubes and Foley catheters are placed as indicated.

DEFINITIVE CARE

When the secondary survey is completed it should be possible to plan definitive treatment. Immediate life-threatening issues have been dealt with, and all the trauma-related problems have been documented and can be properly prioritized and then referred to appropriate specialists for management. Keep in mind that the key features of the Advanced Trauma Life Support System protocol are its rapidity, organization, thoroughness, and hierarchy so that immediately life-threatening issues are identified and treated first.

B
APPENDIX

Measuring Compartment Pressures

Any physician caring for orthopaedic patients must know how to measure a compartment pressure. These measurements may determine whether a patient will require emergency fasciotomy to prevent worsening of compartmental ischemia. Although the development of compartment syndrome is usually diagnosed through the history and physical exam, compartment pressure measurements will help to confirm the diagnosis (and distinguish the condition from neurapraxia or arterial occlusion). Being able to measure compartment pressures accurately and quickly will help you save compromised extremities from irreversible damage or amputation.

THE WHITESIDES TECHNIQUE

The most basic way to measure compartment pressure is a technique described by Whitesides in 1975. Although miniaturized electronic devices have since been developed to make pressure measurement simpler, it is good to know the original Whitesides technique because some hospitals may not have the modern pressure-measuring devices in stock. When you need to measure a compartment pressure, you don't have time to call a company representative and wait for him or her to deliver the device the next day. Muscle necrosis can occur within 6 hours of developing a compartment syndrome, so even an hour's delay in making the diagnosis should be avoided if at all possible. The Whitesides technique requires a few simple components that every emergency room will have. If you know how to measure compartment pressures with a few basic items, you will never compromise care by having to wait for equipment.

The Whitesides technique requires the following equipment:

- A mercury manometer (used to measure blood pressures)
- Plastic IV extension tubing
- A 20-cc Luer-Lok syringe
- Several 18-gauge, 1¼-inch needles
- A four-way stopcock

The basic idea is to draw a small amount of sterile saline into the IV tubing, which has a needle on one end. The other end of the tube, which contains air, is connected to the four-way stopcock. The stopcock serves as a connector that has a 20-cc syringe attached to one port (filled with air) and the mercury manometer connected to another port (connected via another piece of IV extension tubing). This construct is diagrammed in Figures B–1 and B–2. The stopcock is adjusted so that all three ports involved are confluent. To measure a compartment pressure, the needle is placed into the extremity compartment in question (after a skin prep). Next, the syringe plunger is gently pushed forward while observing the small amount of saline in the tubing. While the pressure generated by the syringe plunger is less than that represented by the mercury column in the manometer, the saline bubble will not move and the mercury column will rise in the manometer. As soon as the compartment pressure is less than the plunger force, the saline bubble will start to move toward the extremity. As soon as this occurs, the clinician can simply read off the manometer how high the mercury column has traveled (in millimeters), and that's equal to the compartment pressure. For example, if the saline starts to move towards the extremity when the mercury

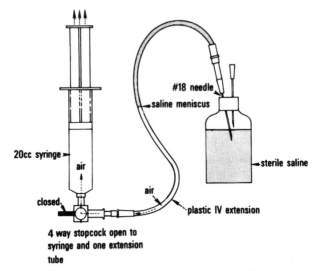

Figure B–1. Initial equipment setup for the Whitesides technique of measuring compartment pressure. (Adapted from Whitesides, TE, Jr, et al: Tissue pressure measurements as a determinant for the need of fasciotomy. Clin Orthop 113:43, 1975, p 45.)

column is 35 mm high, the compartment pressure is 35 mm of mercury.

Although the Whitesides technique is simple to assemble and perform, it helps to have a picture available. The necessary equipment can usually be found in any emergency room, but if a four-way stopcock cannot be found quickly, the next place to look is the intensive care unit.

OTHER TECHNIQUES

Several companies now provide compact devices that further simplify the process of measuring compartment pressure. One such device, manufactured by Stryker Inc., is very simple and reliable. The main unit is about

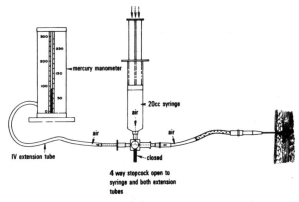

Figure B–2. Compartment pressure is measured by gently depressing the syringe plunger. When pressure within the Whitesides system just exceeds pressure within the extremity, the air bubble in the extension tubing will start moving toward the extremity. At this exact moment, the mercury manometer can be read to yield the compartment pressure. (Adapted from Whitesides, TE, Jr, et al. Tissue pressure measurements as a determinant for the need of fasciotomy. Clin Orthop 113:43, 1975, p 46.)

the size of a deck of cards and comes with a prepackaged fluid-filled cartridge and a long needle. The cartridge snaps inside the main-unit housing, and then the needle is attached to a port on the device. One button "zeros" the device, and then the needle is introduced into the desired compartment. Once this is done, a second button may be pressed, which then provides a digital readout of the pressure. The entire device is lightweight, easy to manipulate, and snaps together in a few seconds.

Another way to measure compartment pressures uses an arterial line setup. Although this is less reliable than the other methods noted above, it can be used to get a rough idea of compartment pressure. The emergency room or intensive care unit nurses can provide you with a pressure reading unit that is used for monitoring arterial lines; all that's necessary then is to place the needle into the compartment and take a reading from the A-line transducer.

GENERAL ADVICE

No matter how the pressure measurements are obtained, a few general points are worth reviewing. First, to prevent making a critical decision based upon one bad number, *take several readings* carefully and make sure they correlate. Leaning against the extremity or mishandling any of the equipment, for example, might produce an aberrant reading that is dramatically too high or too low.

It may be tempting to inject a small amount of local anesthetic into the extremity just before you take a reading. The needle used to take measurements is typically an 18-gauge, and it hurts to have this done without using local anesthetic. *If you do inject a little local anesthetic,* however, *be careful to place it just beneath the skin* so that the local anesthetic itself doesn't inadvertently get into the compartment and thereby further elevate the pressure there.

When dealing with a potentially compromised extremity, be certain not only to take several readings per compartment, but also to *measure several compartments.* In the forearm, for example, three compartments (dorsal, volar, and deep volar) should be checked. Even if the clinical picture of compartment syndrome is obvious, it can be difficult to determine which particular compartment is involved. Be as thorough as possible so that an ischemic zone is not missed.

Document the checking of compartment pressures carefully in the patient's chart. Include what the date and time of the procedure were, where the pressures were checked, what technique was used, and what the pressures were. It is a good idea also to call the orthopaedic attending physician and *directly report your findings.* The decision whether to continue observation or proceed to fasciotomy is a critical one that the attending physician will usually make. As a general guideline, many surgeons will proceed to fasciotomy if the pressure is higher than 30 or 40 mm Hg. There are a variety of published opinions as to what is the critical threshold for compartment pressure, however. Some authors have suggested that the key value is when the pressure is within 30 mm or less of the patient's diastolic blood pressure. For this reason, it is helpful to note the patient's blood pressure when you check the compartment pressure. Many orthopaedic attendings weigh the patient's clinical presentation heavily in deciding how to interpret compartment pressures if the values are borderline. Just remember to document the numbers carefully and discuss them immediately with the orthopaedic attending.

C

Neurologic Assessment

Accurate documentation of a patient's neurologic status is a critical feature of the orthopaedic exam. This appendix reviews five topics that are helpful when recording a patient's motor and sensory function:

1. **Sensory distribution by nerve root level:** Figure C–1 illustrates a sensory map of the body based upon spinal cord root levels. This is also called a *sensory dermatome map.*
2. **Motor function by nerve root level:** Motor function can be graded according to six gradations of strength:

   - Grade 5 ("normal") indicates complete range of motion against gravity with full resistance.
   - Grade 4 ("good") indicates complete range of motion against gravity, but only against moderate or some resistance.
   - Grade 3 ("fair") indicates complete range of motion against gravity with no additional resistance.
   - Grade 2 ("poor") indicates complete range of motion only if gravity is eliminated.
   - Grade 1 ("trace" strength) indicates slight contractility but no active joint motion.
   - Grade 0 indicates no contractility or motion at all.

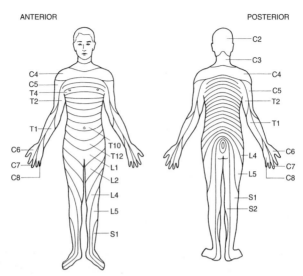

Figure C–1. The sensory dermatomes. (From Nolan, MF: Introduction to the Neurologic Examination. Philadelphia, FA Davis, 1996, p 167, with permission.)

Table C–1 reviews motor function and deep tendon reflexes. This table is not intended to be comprehensive; note that the muscles listed for particular nerve roots are certainly not the only muscles supplied by those roots. In fact, many muscle actions have several nerve root contributions. However, this table does provide a simplified guide that can facilitate a quick assessment of nerve root function by examining the muscles and reflexes noted. For more detailed information, read the *Orthopaedic Neurology* book listed in Appendix F.

3. **Sensory distribution by peripheral nerves:** Table C–2 notes specific areas of the extremities that can be examined to document peripheral nerve sensory function. Again, this table is not a comprehensive listing, but rather a list of areas that generally have a dedicated sensory supply by a specific peripheral nerve. In some individuals, sensory distribution can vary from what is usually accepted as the norm.

Table C–1. MOTOR FUNCTION AND DEEP TENDON REFLEXES

Nerve Root	Muscle to Test	Muscle Action	Deep Tendon Reflex
C5	Deltoid	Shoulder abduction	Biceps
C6	ECRL and ECU	Wrist extension	Brachioradialis
C7	FCR and FCU and EDC	Wrist flexion and finger extension	Triceps
C8	FDS and FDP	Finger flexion	—
T1	Dorsal interossei	Finger abduction	—
T12, L1, L2, L3	Iliopsoas	Hip flexion	—
L2, L3, L4	Quadriceps	Knee extension	—
L2, L3, L4	Adductor brevis, adductor longus, adductor magnus	Hip adduction	—
L4	Tibialis anterior	Foot inversion	Patellar
L5	EDL and EHL	Great and lesser toe extension	—
S1	Peroneus longus and brevis	Foot eversion	Achilles

ECRL = extensor carpi radialis longus; ECU = extensor carpi ulnaris; FCR = flexor carpi radialis; FCU = flexor carpi ulnaris; EDC = extensor digitorum communis, FDS = flexor digitorum superficialis; FDP = flexor digitorum profundus; EDL = extensor digitorum longus; EHL = extensor hallucis longus.

Table C–2. DOCUMENTING PERIPHERAL NERVE SENSORY FUNCTION

Peripheral Nerve	Sensory Area to Test
Axillary	Lateral proximal arm
Musculocutaneous (lateral antebrachial cutaneous branch)	Lateral forearm
Radial	Dorsal first web space in hand
Median	Radial half of palm of hand
Ulnar	Dorsal aspect of ring and small fingers
Lateral femoral cutaneous	Anterior lateral thigh
Sural	Midportion of calf (posterior leg)
Saphenous	Medial anterior leg
Common peroneal	Lateral anterior leg
Superficial peroneal	Dorsum of foot and ankle
Deep peroneal	Dorsal aspect of great toe/second toe web space
Tibial	Heel
Lateral plantar	Undersurface of forefoot, lateral 1.5 toes
Medial plantar	Undersurface of forefoot, medial 3.5 toes

Table C–3. DOCUMENTING PERIPHERAL NERVE MOTOR FUNCTION

Peripheral Nerve	Motor Function to Test
Radial (proximal to elbow)	Elbow extension
Radial (distal to elbow)	Wrist and thumb extension
Anterior interosseous (branch of median in forearm)	"A-OK" sign: thumb and index interphalangeal joint flexion
Median (at wrist)	Thumb abduction
Ulnar (at wrist)	Finger abduction and adduction
Femoral	Knee extension
Obturator	Hip adduction
Tibial	Knee flexion and toe flexion
Deep peroneal	Ankle and toe dorsiflexion
Superficial peroneal	Foot eversion

**Table C–4. PRESENTATION OF
INCOMPLETE SPINAL CORD
INJURY SYNDROMES**

Spinal Cord Syndrome	Clinical Presentation
Central cord syndrome	The most common incomplete cord injury syndrome. Patients are quadriplegic with sacral sparing. Upper extremities are affected more than lower. Chance of functional recovery is good (75%).
Anterior cord syndrome	Also a common syndrome. Patients demonstrate complete motor deficit, but torso and lower-extremity deep pressure and proprioception are present. Likelihood of functional recovery is low (10%).
Posterior cord syndrome	Relatively rare. Patients show loss of deep pressure, deep pain, and proprioception.
Brown-Séquard's syndrome	More common than posterior cord syndrome but less common than anterior or central cord syndrome. Patients have ipsilateral motor deficit and contralateral loss of pain and temperature perception. Likelihood of recovery is high (>90%).

4. **Motor function by peripheral nerves:** Table C–3 provides a guide for examining the motor function of common peripheral nerves.
5. **Incomplete spinal cord injury syndromes:** Table C–4 summarizes the physical presentation of several well-described incomplete spinal cord injury syndromes.

D

Anesthetic Techniques Suitable for Fracture Manipulation

This appendix reviews several common methods of managing pain during fracture manipulation. Fracture manipulation is much easier to accomplish if the patient is comfortable and relaxed.

HEMATOMA BLOCK

A hematoma block is a workhorse for managing distal radial fractures. It can also be used for other fractures, such as radial and ulnar shaft fractures in children, but its most frequent common application is the distal radius and ulna. The block consists of injecting a small amount of local anesthetic into the fracture hematoma, producing pain relief for fracture manipulation.

The hematoma block works best if the hematoma is fresh, which allows the local anesthetic to mix and bathe the fracture surfaces. If the fracture is more than 24 hours old, the block may not work as well because the hematoma may no longer be particularly fluid. The block sometimes can take 10 or 20 minutes to take maximal effect, so it is often efficient to administer the block first and then spend the next several minutes organizing the equipment needed to reduce the fracture and apply a cast. By the time you're ready to manipulate the patient's wrist and start wrapping cast padding, the block should have had time to take effect. Keep in mind that although a hematoma block works just as well in children as in adults, some children (probably most under the age 8 years) will not tolerate a needle stick into their fracture site, so alternative methods of pain control (i.e., IV or intramuscular routes of pain medication) may be better or additionally required.

The standard agent used is 1% lidocaine (Xylocaine [without epinephrine]). Only about 5 mL is required, and it helps to draw the lidocaine into a 10-cc syringe. Use a 22-gauge needle to inject because this size needle is not large enough to hurt the patient, but it is large enough to withdraw the hematoma and inject anesthetic. Once the lidocaine syringe is ready, prep the patient's skin over the fracture hematoma with a small wipe of iodine solution, and place the needle exactly where you think the fracture hematoma is located. It helps greatly to have the patient's x-rays hanging on a view box in front of you as you inject. Even though the location of the fracture might initially seem obvious, it can occasionally be difficult to immediately find the hematoma. Palpate the wrist gently, glance at the films frequently (the way a golfer eyes the flag while lining up a putt), and then insert the needle. Do not inject the lidocaine yet. Instead, gently draw back on the syringe plunger, looking for dark red blood returning into the syringe. Do not inject until you see this because only this sign means that your needle is in the right place. Fracture hematoma is generally plentiful and under some pressure, so if your needle is there, several milliliters of dark red blood will flash back into your syringe quite easily. Be sure your needle is down to bone (so that you cannot possibly be in a vein), and be certain that the blood return is dark red (not arterial blood). When you are certain that you have penetrated the hematoma, you can slowly start to inject the lidocaine. At this point, the patient will usually complain most of intense pressure at the fracture site, so inject slowly.

Sometimes it is less painful to inject a little, then draw back a little, and then inject a little more, and so on. This eases the intense pressure of adding volume to an already swollen space and also tends to "bathe" the fracture in lidocaine and may help the block take effect.

No more than 5 or 6 mL of lidocaine is necessary. Using too much Xylocaine can produce a risk of Xylocaine toxicity side effects, but a single block with 5 mL of 1% Xylocaine is unlikely to cause any problems, even in children.*

Withdraw the needle and have the patient hold a gauze sponge on the needle site while you ready the plaster cast, because the skin puncture wound will tend to drain Xylocaine and hematoma for a few minutes.

The hematoma block can produce outstanding pain relief, allowing you to manipulate a badly broken distal radial fracture with the patient hardly noticing at all. Be aware, though, that if the distal ulna is also broken (it usually is), in some cases an additional few milliliters of lidocaine may be required at a second site over the ulnar injury to effect a total block. Many times, however, the radial hematoma communicates with the ulnar injury, and both fractures are treated with the same injection. Furthermore, even if the distal ulnar fracture is not affected by the radial injection, it just may not hurt enough to warrant a separate injection.

---

*A few notes about local anesthetic toxicity: Toxicity is additive, so mixing lidocaine and bupivacaine will require reductions in maximum dosing. Toxicity is related to the vascularity of tissues, so subcutaneous injections are less likely to produce side effects than are intravascular injections. It may be helpful to know the maximum safe dosage for lidocaine because it is such a commonly used drug. In adults, a generally accepted upper limit of lidocaine (without epinephrine) is 500 mg and 225 mg for bupivacaine. Another way to estimate lidocaine dosing is about 5 mg of lidocaine per kg of body weight (but no more than 500 mg). Remember that 1% lidocaine contains 10 mg of drug per one milliliter of volume, so that 50 cc of 1% lidocaine would contain 500 mg of drug; 25 cc of 2% lidocaine also contains 500 mg of drug. For the purpose of hematoma block and digital blocks, usually only 5 to 7 cc of 1% lidocaine is required, which is well below the maximal dose. A good rule for administration of local anesthetic is to use as little as necessary.

PERIPHERAL NERVE BLOCK

Direct injection of local anesthetic into subcutaneous tissues around a particular nerve is also a simple and effective pain management technique for certain fractures. A "metacarpal" block is an example of a peripheral nerve block that is very helpful for managing finger fractures or lacerations. Again, 1% lidocaine is the agent of choice; be certain that it does not contain added epinephrine, which could cause digital ischemia if injected at the metacarpal level. A total of 6 mL is needed for a metacarpal block, and a 25-gauge needle is ideal. Inject 3 mL of lidocaine on each side of the affected finger, aiming for the volar web space just adjacent to the metacarpal head. It is usually unnecessary to inject circumferentially around the finger; doing so runs the risk of blocking venous return or producing digital ischemia. The target of the injection in a metacarpal block is the digital nerve on each side of the affected finger, and its location is reliable at the branch point of the common digital nerve, located about 1/2 inch proximal to the web space. If a short (5/8-inch) needle is used, insert the needle all the way to its hub and inject about 3 mL of local anesthetic; repeat on the other side of the affected finger. The block usually works within a few minutes and will provide anesthesia for the finger distal to midproximal phalanx.

This block will not anesthetize the metacarpal head area and is not effective for metacarpal head fractures. Mixing some 0.25% bupivacaine with the lidocaine will extend the efficacy of the block so that it will last several hours instead of just 30 minutes. A typical mixture would be half bupivacaine and half Xylocaine: 3 mL of 1% lidocaine (without epinephrine) and 3 mL of 0.25% bupivacaine (without epinephrine).

INTRAVENOUS OR INTRAMUSCULAR ADMINISTRATION OF MEDICATION

In some situations, IV administration of narcotic and sedative medication is appropriate for fracture care. Usually, these will be situations where a hematoma block or local injection around a nerve is not possible or inadequate. Furthermore, if a particular block is not completely effective, a small amount of IV sedation may be a perfect adjunct. Although the exact doses of medication are beyond the scope of this text, the following general comments may be helpful.

Perhaps the most important point when using IV or intramuscular narcotic (or sedative) is not to overmedicate the patient and risk respiratory arrest. Most institutions require that some monitoring protocol be followed, such as blood pressure measurements and pulse oximetry. You should also be in an environment where immediate respiratory support and full cardiopulmonary resuscitation capabilities are available (e.g., the emergency room). Reversal agents, such as naloxone (Narcan), should be handy. Using IV or intramuscular sedation for a procedure at the patient's bedside on the inpatient floor is asking for trouble.

Start administering the narcotic or sedation with small amounts first and see how the patient reacts. Sometimes just a little medication is required to achieve the desired effect, especially in elderly patients and young children. If intramuscular narcotic is used, be sure to allow enough time to pass (sometimes 30 or 45 minutes) for the medication to take effect. Attempting to manipulate a radial and ulnar shaft fracture only 5 minutes after intramuscular narcotic has been given is not likely to be a satisfying experience.

E
APPENDIX

Glossary of Fracture Terminology

Angulation. A bending alignment between two bone fragments. "Ninety degrees angulated" means the two bone fragments are perpendicular.

Bayonet apposition. A type of fracture position that is characterized by 100% displacement of the bone ends and shortening. One bone end is completely on top of the other, and the overall length has been reduced because the two bones can slide toward each other.

Butterfly fragment. A triangular piece of bone that occurs in long-bone shaft fractures. This fragment is a distinct piece, separate from the proximal and distal shaft segments. A fracture with a butterfly fragment requires more energy to create than a simple two-part transverse or oblique fracture.

Callus. New bone formation that occurs as a fracture heals. Fracture callus initially appears disorganized and cloudlike; as the fracture heals, it becomes more dense and organized.

Colles's fracture. Named after Abraham Colles, this is a fracture of the distal radius that technically involves only the metaphyseal portion of the bone and does not extend to the articular surface. The distal fragment is volarly angulated and dorsally displaced relative to the proximal segment.

Comminuted fracture. A fracture with more than two or three pieces. Comminution usually means that higher energy was involved in producing the fracture, which created a "shattered" type of appearance, with many small fragments and secondary fracture lines.

Diaphysis. The shaft area of a long bone. This region is usually the narrowest area of the bone and has thick cortical margins. The narrowest part of the diaphysis is called the *isthmus*.

Diastasis. A nonlongitudinal gap between fracture fragments. Significant diastasis of fracture fragments that comprise a joint surface usually requires correction to reduce the likelihood of developing posttraumatic arthritis.

Displacement. The degree to which two fracture fragments are touching each other. For example, a femoral shaft fracture that is 50% displaced means that the two ends of the broken femur are translated away from each other so that only 50% of the distal portion is touching the proximal fracture fragment.

Distraction. A longitudinal gap between fracture fragments. For example, applying too much traction to a fracture can produce distraction at the fracture site. Sometimes soft tissue (muscle or tendon, for example) can become entrapped in a fracture and produce distraction of the major fragments.

Epiphysis. The area of a long bone that is between the physis (growth plate) and nearest end of the bone.

Greenstick fracture. A type of fracture that occurs in children, usually in the shafts of the forearm bones. The cortex on one side of the bone is broken, but the other side is intact, the way a fresh ("green") tree branch might break. The bone has a bent appearance. Greenstick fractures are characteristic of children because the periosteum around the cortex is very thick, and the bone cortex is more rubbery in character. An adult bone is more brittle, and if bent too far, will snap in two like a dry branch.

Impacted. Typical of crush-type fractures in which a fracture segment is jammed down into the proximal segment. A depression-type deformity results relative to the normal geometry of the bone.

Isthmus. The narrowest part of the diaphysis.

Metaphysis. The area of a long bone between the shaft of the bone (diaphysis) and growth plate. The metaphysis typically flares out in diameter so that it is wider than the shaft region of the bone. The metaphyseal area usually has thinner cortical bone margins and a broader area of cancellous bone.

Oblique fracture. Similar to a spiral fracture but usually shorter in length. The fracture line makes a more acute angle relative to the perpendicular axis of the bone (and doesn't travel completely around the shaft of the bone, as in a spiral fracture).

Physis. A cartilaginous zone present in skeletally immature bone, which is responsible for longitudinal bone growth. On x-ray, the physis appears to be a radiolucent line that can be confused with a transverse fracture. The Salter-Harris classification organizes fractures involving the physis into five types. The physis is also sometimes referred to as the *growth plate*. The physes of long bones are located very close to either end of the bone.

Pilon. A specific type of fracture in the distal tibia that results from an axial load. This fracture often requires surgery if any malalignment is present because it represents an intra-articular fracture of the ankle joint, and posttraumatic arthritis may develop unless near-perfect alignment is achieved.

Plastic deformation. A type of injury in which the shaft of bone is bent but not actually broken. A greenstick fracture has one cortex broken and one cortex intact; the plastically deformed bone has neither cortex broken. This injury occurs typically in children (thick periosteum equals "rubbery" bones) and can produce a significant angulatory deformity of the limb.

Rotation. The twisting of two fracture fragments with respect to each other around a common longitudinal axis. "Malrotation of 90 degrees" indicates that the two fragments are twisted 90 degrees out of normal alignment with respect to each other.

Shortening. Overlapping or settling of a fracture that produces an overall smaller total bone length than normal.

Spiral fracture. A fracture line that rotates around the shaft of the bone, typically traveling several bone diameters in length. This type of fracture is often produced by twisting forces acting on the bone.

Torus fracture. A buckle fracture, common in small children. An axial load produces this injury. The bone fails on one side and wrinkles into a shortened state.

Transverse fracture. A fracture line that is perpendicular to the long axis of the bone.

Valgus. An angulatory deformity, or bend in the bone, as seen from an anteroposterior view. The apex of the bend points *towards* the midline of the body.

Varus. An angulatory deformity, or bend in the bone, as seen from an anteroposterior view. The apex of the bend points *away* from the midline of the body.

F
APPENDIX

Suggested Reading

GENERAL REVIEW

Orthopaedic Knowledge Update (OKU)

This outstanding text is a supercondensed "bible" of contemporary orthopaedic clinical and basic science. It is published every 3 years by the American Academy of Orthopaedic Surgeons (AAOS) and is read by orthopaedic surgeons throughout the country as a way of keeping current in the field. It includes a topic-oriented suggested reading list at the end of each chapter. This is a *must* for orthopaedic trainees.

Journal of the American Academy of Orthopaedic Surgeons (JAAOS)

Published six times per year by the AAOS, this publication has the largest orthopaedic journal readership in the country. It is a superbly edited collection of contemporary review articles and is another *"must-read"* source for orthopaedic trainees and attendings alike.

Instructional Course Lectures

This is a yearly AAOS publication that covers about half a dozen general topics in every volume. Each topic is covered by a series of 3 to 10 articles that are specifically selected for their clarity and organization, written by nationally recognized experts. The Instructional Course Lectures are widely recognized as another outstanding contemporary review source.

Review of Orthopaedics

By Mark D. Miller, M.D. (W.B. Saunders, Philadelphia, 1998, 2nd ed, 372 pp).
This review manual is a well-organized and detailed collection of clinical and basic science facts.

FRACTURE TEXTBOOKS

Rockwood, CA, Jr, et al (eds): ***Rockwood & Green's Fractures in Adults,*** ed 4 (3 vols). Lippincott-Raven, Philadelphia, 1996, 4100 pp.

Rockwood, CA, Jr, et al (eds): ***Fractures in Children,*** ed 4. Lippincott-Raven, Philadelphia, 1996, 1232 pp.

These are widely recognized as the definitive reference texts for fracture care.

Browner, BD, et al (Edited by Richard Lampert): ***Skeletal Trauma: Fractures, Dislocations, Ligamentous Injuries,*** ed 2 (2 vols). WB Saunders, Philadelphia, 1997, 2400 pp.

Green, NE, and Swiontkowski, MF (Edited by Richard Lampert): ***Skeletal Trauma in Children,*** ed 2. WB Saunders, Philadelphia, 1997, 608 pp.

Another comprehensive and well-written reference text.

Mueller, ME, et al: ***The Manual of Internal Fixation,*** ed 3. Springer-Verlag, New York, 1995, 750 pp.

This is the definitive text for the AO techniques of fracture care, written by the Swiss surgeons who refined and popularized these methods. In addition to a comprehensive discussion of operative fracture management, the book includes a detailed review of fracture biology and AO instrumentation.

GUIDE TO PHYSICAL EXAMINATION

Hoppenfeld, S: *Physical Examination of the Spine and Extremities.* Appleton & Lange, Norwalk, Conn, 1976, 276 pp.
Although the book may initially appear to be a collection of cartoons, it is perhaps one of the best-written texts concerning the orthopaedic physical exam. Serious orthopaedic trainees should commit this text to memory.

Hoppenfeld, S: *Orthopaedic Neurology: A Diagnostic Guide to Neurologic Levels.* Lippincott-Raven, Philadelphia, 1977, 131 pp.
Somewhat shorter than the previous book but just as outstanding, this text reviews the neurology that orthopaedists should know. This book also belongs stored in your memory bank.

MAJOR JOURNALS

The journals noted subsequently are good for topic-oriented or author-specific research. The following list is only a limited sampling of what's available in the peer-review literature:

The Journal of Bone and Joint Surgery
Clinical Orthopaedics and Related Research
The Journal of Pediatric Orthopaedics
The Journal of Hand Surgery
Foot and Ankle
Spine
Arthroscopy and Arthroscopically Related Surgery

Index

Page numbers followed by an "f" indicate figures; page numbers followed by a "t" indicate tabular material.